Doping in Non-Olympic Sports

This book is the first of its kind to discuss doping within Non-Olympic Sports. Sports like American football, cricket, and dance sports have, in recent years, been in the news for doping activities. The scale of the incidents may differ in each of these sports, but they present interesting questions about the legitimacy of the World Anti-Doping Agency (WADA) Code.

Doping in Non-Olympic Sports: Challenging the Legitimacy of WADA? argues against the International Olympic Committee (IOC)-run regime where WADA Code compliance is used as the only parameter to define an activity as a sport. This book argues that the definition of modern sport is based on certain factors identified through sociological and historical research. These parameters are common across the board and do not distinguish between Olympic and Non-Olympic sports. However, the use of the word Olympic in the Non-Olympic sport terminology subjects such sports to IOC dictates. Consequently, the IOC exploits its monopoly over the word Olympics to insist on WADA Code compliances. The numerous instances of doping, as reported, go on to prove that WADA is turning a blind eye to these Non-Olympic sports.

This book is the first to dissect the issue of doping within Non-Olympic sports and questions the very idea of WADA compliance as a condition precedent to defining sports going on to highlight the inbuilt inequity within the existing anti-doping system wherein a private regime is usurping the State's discretion. The new, cutting-edge research book is key reading for academics and researchers in the fields of Coaching, Sports Pharmacology, Sports Medicine, Sports Law, and the related disciplines.

Lovely Dasgupta is Associate Professor of Law at the West Bengal National University of Juridical Sciences, India, with particular interests in Sports Law, Competition Law, and Contract Law. She became one of the pioneers in the field of studying and researching Sports Law from an Indian perspective and was one of the first from the Indian legal fraternity to develop and teach the subject called Sports Law.

Routledge Research in Sport, Culture and Society

For more information about this series, please visit: www.routledge.com/sport/series/RRSCS

Doping in Non-Olympic Sports

Challenging the Legitimacy of WADA?

Lovely Dasgupta

R Routledge
Taylor & Francis Group

NEW YORK AND LONDON

First published 2022
by Routledge
605 Third Avenue, New York, NY 10158

and by Routledge
2 Park Square, Milton Park, Abingdon, Oxon, OX14 4RN

Routledge is an imprint of the Taylor & Francis Group, an informa business

Library of Congress Cataloging-in-Publication Data
A catalog record for this book has been requested

ISBN: 978-0-367-53514-8 (hbk)
ISBN: 978-0-367-56018-8 (pbk)
ISBN: 978-1-003-08230-9 (ebk)

DOI: 10.4324/9781003082309

Typeset in Times New Roman
by Apex CoVantage, LLC

Contents

1 Prologue

This book is the first to dissect the issue of doping within Non-Olympic sports. Non-Olympic sports encompass those sports that are recognized by the IOC but are not included in the Olympic Games. The process of recognition of an International Federation is detailed out in the Olympic Charter. Hence even if a sport is not included in the Olympic Games, it can be given recognition. The grant of recognition is, however, subject to the requirement of WADA compliance. In short, if an IF is in the list of the recognized federation, there is a presumption that the IF will be strictly complying with the WADA Code. Unfortunately, the reality is far removed from the idyllic picture that the IOC would want us to believe. The 2015 report of Al Jazeera, an outcome of investigative journalism, showed the connivance of sports stars with the doping mafia. Big names like Peyton Manning, the legendary quarter back of NFL, were alleged to have used HGH. The report revealed that laboratories in US supplied PEDs to the NFL star and others. Notwithstanding the challenge to the said report, in the US courts, it does indicate the prevalence of doping in American football. Instances of doping in NFL are often talked about and definitely is a matter of concern. Though the USA Federation of American Football (USFAF) deals with amateur sports, it is equally complacent on doping issues. In May 2017, the International Federation of American Football (IFAF) had suspended the membership of the US Federation of American Football (USFAF) for anti-doping violations. Yet, the poor record on anti-doping measures has not affected the popularity of NFL or American football across the globe. Nor did the revelations of the Al Jazeera report affect the popularity of Peyton Manning for he retains his status as an iconic personality.

That doping scandals hardly matter within Non-Olympic sports holds equally true in the case of cricket. Though the International Cricket Council (ICC) has on paper signed up WADA, the track record of some of its powerful National Association is nothing to write home about. The Board of Cricket Control of India (BCCI), for instance, has vehemently opposed the WADA Code. This opposition has not affected the popularity of cricket or the cricketers. Doping incidences are under-reported. Further sanctions, if imposed, are mild and appear to be tokenism. Interestingly, corruption in cricket in the form of match-fixing and betting is a well-documented affair. Though doping hardly

DOI: 10.4324/9781003082309-1

appears to be a debatable issue, the cricketers go about their business without any fear. Another glaring example of rampant PED abuse in a Non-Olympic sport is Dance sport. Studies conducted to understand doping in Dance sport go on to prove the same. WADA's report on anti-doping rule violation in the fringe sports lists Dance sport as one of the biggest offenders. This has, however, not deprived Dance sport of the patronage of IOC or WADA. These examples establish doping as an integral aspect of Non-Olympic sports. Importantly, lax anti-doping measures have not affected the adulation of the spectators for these sports. This fact posits an interesting question as to the legitimacy of the WADA Code. Importantly neither ICC nor IFAF and nor World Dance Sport Federation (WDSF) has been derecognized because one of their members or few of their players are going scot-free or let off with lesser punishment.

De-recognition appears to be a harsh punishment for incidences of doping though the same is not unprecedented. Russia, being the biggest example, is under threat to be banned from Tokyo 2020. Further, the recognition of Non-Olympic sports by IOC has no rationale except that it makes good business sense. The IOC gets to include the sport at a later stage in the Olympic Games. It also helps IOC to expand its network among various groups and communities within different countries. Thus, Non-Olympic sports ambivalence on anti-doping measures does not appear to be a problem. Importantly, the IOC appears to be satisfied with compliances in form rather than substances. Being a signatory of the WADA Code is enough, the actual compliances with WADA Code do not appear to be a matter of concern for IOC or WADA. This ready recognition of a Non-Olympic sport, based on formal compliances, thus creates a problem within the existing anti-doping regime. At one end are the elite Olympic sports, wherein the athletes are under tremendous pressure to strictly follow the WADA Code or perish. The livelihood of athletes is jeopardized due to the excessive burden of proof, under the current anti-doping regime.

The athletes are under constant scrutiny, and compliances level are high and taxing both mentally and financially. On the other hand, within the Non-Olympic sports, business goes on as usual for the athletes despite innumerable instances of doping. The only concern of the athletes from Non-Olympic sports is to perform and not get bogged down by substantive compliances. There is hardly any long-drawn litigation nor are high-profile sanctions being imposed. This book looks into this dichotomy and questions the rationale of the current anti-doping regime. This book argues that accommodation of inconsistencies in the WADA Code compliances undermines the legitimacy of the anti-doping regime. Moreover, such inconsistencies are unfair to athletes practicing the Olympic sports, and they have to bear the entire brunt of the strict liability doctrine. For the WADA Code to be truly inclusive, IOC has to ensure that compliances are substantive. Further, the exemptions and exceptions need to be worked out not based on an International Federations bargaining power but based on the legitimate needs of sports. Accordingly, both IOC and WADA need to play a more proactive role in identifying the sports they want to recognize and then help these federations in complying with the

WADA Code. Burdening the States Governments with the responsibility of WADA Code compliances does not work in the case of developing and poor countries. Further, since the prerogative of recognition or de-recognition is within the domain of IOC, the responsibility has to be that of IOC. WADA Code compliance being a condition precedent to the process of recognition, WADA has also to take the responsibility.

Themes

WADA Code forms the bedrock of the current anti-doping regime, which is being accepted and followed stringently across the world. The sporting world being a hierarchical setup has ensured that the athletes are bereft of all choices vis-à-vis the system they will follow. WADA Code is the first and the last resort for anyone planning to take sports as a source of livelihood. Sports, as we understand, is usually thought in terms of Olympic sports. However, the cultural, political, social, and legal factors also impact the definition of sports. This reality is best exemplified by the Tokyo 2020 sports list. Tokyo 2020 has included baseball/softball, karate, skateboarding, sport climbing, and surfing based on their popularity among the Japanese population. These sports are thus included for enhancing the marketability of the Olympics. Prior to their inclusion in the Tokyo 2020, these sports belonged to the category of Non-Olympic sports. This book identifies the important role that IOC and WADA play in creating the list of Non-Olympic sports. This book re-affirms the hegemony that IOC has over everything sports. This automatically brings WADA into the discussion. This book questions the very idea of WADA compliance as a condition precedent to defining sports. The idea of sports has to be delinked from IOC and its institutions for the determination of what is sports has different considerations. As the studies by sociologists and sports historians have revealed that modern sport across the board is about records and statistics.

The anti-doping rhetoric within sports is well established; however, this book brings into focus the absence of any literature on doping in Non-Olympic sports. Considering that almost all the Non-Olympic sports have adopted WADA Code, this appears to be a missing link. An understanding of this scenario is needed to test the efficacy as well as the viability of the current WADA Code. A review of reported incidents of doping in Non-Olympic sports reveals that American football, baseball, and cricket lead the list of suspects. Considering that baseball is now to be part of the Tokyo 2020 Games, this book zeros down on American football and cricket. Dance sport is also discussed primarily to outline that the doping problem appears to exist both in mainstream Non-Olympic sports and in fringe Non-Olympic sports. This book further establishes that the problem of doping within Non-Olympic sports has the same contours as in Olympic sports. Thus, the lack of literature is not evidence of a lack of doping in these sports.

This book finally tries to highlight the inbuilt inequity within the existing anti-doping system wherein a private regime is usurping the State's discretion.

Both WADA and IOC are exceeding their mandate by burdening the States with the responsibility of WADA compliances. In the case of Olympic sports, the imposition is understandable as part of the trade-off. However, vis-à-vis Non-Olympic sports, such impositions are not acceptable. This book argues that there lacks a legal basis for such impositions since in many cases the State themselves do not fund the Non-Olympic sports. For Non-Olympic sports by being outside the Olympic Games are not bound by Olympism or WADA Code. Doping in Non-Olympic sports then needs to be understood purely from the health of the athlete's perspective. Further, the adoption of the WADA Code needs to be a voluntary act of the Non-Olympic sports federations. And, the driving force for such adoption should be a conviction that the WADA Code provides the best set of anti-doping regulations. Importantly, Non-Olympic sports should be allowed to customize their anti-doping program as per their requirements. In case States do fund the Non-Olympic sports, they can insist on WADA Code compliance as part of their domestic law or policy. Accordingly, these concerns are presented in the form of five chapters, each one putting forth the anti-doping narrative within the Non-Olympic sports.

Chapter 2 initiates the discussion by pointing out that the recognition of a sport by the International Olympic Committee (hereinafter IOC) is preconditioned upon, among others, the WADA Code compliance. The question, however, is: how is the WADA Code compliance to be judged? Further, recognition does not mean that the sport will automatically be part of the grand spectacle called the Olympic Games. The recognition of an International Federation, however, is the first step toward getting admitted to the hallowed halls of the Olympics. The sport gets the chance to be called an Olympic sport. The athletes/players get the chance to win Olympic medals and bask in the Olympic glory. The Olympic Charter is the document that lays down the foundation for such recognition by the IOC. Unfortunately, though the Charter is completely silent as to the process of granting such recognition. The only thing that appears to be clear is the fact that the ultimate arbiter of such a decision is the IOC. The dominance of IOC means that the designation of an activity as a sporting activity is ambiguous. It depends on the whims and fancies of the IOC. Interestingly, the criteria for recognition of a sport are, however, the same across the board. The uniform standard appears equitable but it creates problems at two levels. At the level of compliance postrecognition, there is a clear disparity between the Olympic sports and the Non-Olympic sports. The sports persons are subjected to different standards of scrutiny and regulations depending upon the level of performance. The sports persons/athletes participating in the Olympics are required to undergo rigorous tests, as part of the WADA Code compliance. The athletes/sports persons, as part of the Olympic sports, are constantly under the spotlight. Hence, their actions are regularly scrutinized for determining rule violations. On the other hand, Non-Olympic sports persons/athletes fall under the radar. The level of scrutiny that they are subjected to is minimal. They neither have to bear the rigors of the system nor are they living under the fear of constant threat to career and livelihood.

The present system creates two different worlds within sports. It dilutes the importance of the WADA Code since Non-Olympic sports are granted recognition by satisfying only the formal criteria. There is no compulsion or process that ensures substantive compliances. This chapter questions the very model adopted by the IOC to grant recognition. It questions the rationale of insisting on WADA compliance. It begins by analyzing and surveying the Olympic system. This chapter highlights the various processes that are involved before a sport gains recognition by IOC. It looks into the consequence of being an IOC-recognized sport. and the role of WADA in the entire process of recognition. It analyzes the WADA Code (both 2015 and 2021) to understand as well as explains the impact of the Code on the process of recognition. It compares the compliance level of the Non-Olympic sport with the Olympic sport. This chapter concludes by arguing that WADA Code compliance need not be the pre-condition for grant of recognition to a sport.

In Chapter 3, inquiries are made into the prevalence of doping within American football and the role played by the International Federation of American Football (IFAF). American football presents a peculiar instance within the narrative on Non-Olympic sports. The sport is split into amateur and professional. And the trajectory of anti-doping compliances within the two is equally divergent. The sport presents a compelling study into the effectiveness of the World Anti-Doping Agency (WADA) Code and its anti-doping program. Importantly, this chapter builds upon the argument professed in the previous chapter, viz., there is laxity in enforcement of anti-doping program within the Non-Olympic sports. American football is a good example to substantiate the above point. The sport has faced criticism for its lax attitude toward anti-doping enforcements. However, the same does not seem to have any effect. This chapter begins by introducing the two ends of this sport, viz., amateur and professional football and analyzes the anti-doping trajectory within these two ends. A comparison is made between the anti-doping measures within the professional sphere and its amateur counterpart. This chapter then goes onto analyzing the anti-doping cases, as reported in the media and debated before the Court of Arbitration for Sports (CAS). The tussle between the USA and other members of IFAF on anti-doping measures is discussed herein. This chapter then goes onto critique the criterion that WADA and International Olympic Committee (IOC) had applied for granting recognition to IFAF and looks into the role of the WADA and the IOC in view of lapses by IFAF in effective enforcement of the Code. This chapter also inspects the interrelationship between NFL and IFAF and the anti-doping narrative they both support and promote. This chapter argues that IFAF and NFL anti-doping controversies challenge the homogenization process of WADA. Finally, this chapter insists that the continued recognition of IFAF and the relatively benign reaction of both IOC and WADA have everything to do with the bargaining power of the members.

In Chapter 4, the problem of doping in cricket is looked into. The International Cricket Council (ICC) is the governing body of cricket. Considering that the sports have a huge fan following in some of the world's most populous regions, its stand on doping merits attention. This chapter thus analyzes the anti-doping program of the ICC. It begins by analyzing the implementation of the World Anti-Doping Agency (WADA) by the ICC. This will facilitate understanding the compliance level of the ICC vis-à-vis the WADA Code. This chapter deals with the approach of the ICC's members in dealing with doping allegations within the sport. This will help understand the equation of the ICC with its members on the issue of WADA Code compliance. Importantly, it will establish the extent to which ICC is serious in dealing with doping. Further, it will also explain the efforts of the ICC in ensuring effective compliance with the WADA Code. It will also help in understanding the consequence that the individual members are likely to face in defying the diktat of ICC. It will also help understand the reasons that convinced International Olympic Committee (IOC) to grant recognition to ICC. ICC's anti-doping measures will also help understand its philosophy as a Non-Olympic sport. Considering that Non-Olympic sports, in general, have been lax toward WADA Code compliance, this understanding is important. This chapter then analyzes in detail the equation of ICC with the Board of Control for Cricket in India (BCCI). This study is important since currently BCCI dominates the sport. Hence, it is indeed a powerful member of the ICC. Therefore, the approach of BCCI toward implementation of the WADA Code is relevant and necessary. It is relevant because BCCI's attitude toward the ICC's anti-doping program determines the narrative on the issue. It is necessary for understanding the control of ICC over BCCI. These analyses will also help us understand the effectiveness of the overall governance structure of ICC. It is also relevant in determining the steps that the IOC ought to take to force ICC to enforce the WADA Code stringently. This chapter will also look into the response of the World Anti-Doping Agency (WADA) toward BCCI's anti-doping program. This is needed to understand the bargaining powers that are involved herein. Accordingly, one needs to look into the bargaining power of ICC as a Non-Olympic sport vis-à-vis the IOC. Similarly, the bargaining power of ICC vis-à-vis WADA is looked into. The same is done to understand the key factors that lead to the adoption of the WADA Code by the ICC. Analysis on similar lines is made to understand the bargaining power that exists between the ICC and the BCCI. The attempt is to understand the conflict area that exists between the ICC and BCCI on the issues of WADA Code compliance. This chapter argues that the ICC versus BCCI tussle on anti-doping measure is an instance of power play. This chapter points out that to access large markets of South Asia, both WADA and IOC continue to ignore the lax anti-doping measures of ICC. The ICC needs BCCI for its existence; hence, the power play here too is based on the bargaining power of the members.

Chapter 5 deals with a sport that is not regarded as such. Dance sport does not invoke the images of doping; however, it does have a serious problem in this area. There are empirical researches done, which highlight the prevalence of substance abuse and doping in Dance sport. This chapter takes up the sport primarily because of its uniqueness. For not many would consider Dance as a sport. Further, Dance sport is different from other sports primarily because it is a generic term that includes different forms of dance within its ambit. Last, Dance sport has been in the public sphere for long and accordingly has also got the attention of the International Olympic Committee (IOC). Accordingly, Dance sport is one of the oldest recognized Non-Olympic sports. Despite the length for which Dance sport has enjoyed the status of a Non-Olympic sport, it has yet to join the Olympic program. Another factor that needs to be analyzed is the process of recognition of Dance sport as a Non-Olympic sport. This is so because of the relatively easier terms and conditions that prevailed at the time when Dance sport was recognized by IOC. The time when Dance sport got recognition, there was no compulsion to have a robust anti-doping program in place. Accordingly, the parameters of recognition were not focused on this aspect of the governance of the sport. Dance sport comparatively had it easy in terms of getting recognized as a Non-Olympic sport. Another interesting bit about Dance sport is the multiplicity of Governing Bodies (GB) that were initially in charge of the sport. The body recognized by the IOC is different from the current organization in charge of Dance sport. And that calls for an interesting study into Dance sport as a Non-Olympic sport. Considering that it continues to campaign for inclusion in the Olympic program, the claim needs to be tested. This chapter begins by analyzing the evolution of Dance from Art to sport. The process through which the sport went on to achieve its current form as a Non-Olympic sport will be reviewed. The governance issues led to the multiple changes of guard within the administrative structure of the Dance sport. Next this chapter looks at the prevalence of doping within dance sport. The chapter investigates the anti-doping program that the IF, currently in charge of the sport, enforces. The analyses includes a study of the rules and regulations that are used to enforce the anti-doping program. The analyses involve the study of the impact that compliance requirement within the WADA Code is likely to have on a relatively small International Federation. Importantly, the WADA Code compliance issue with Dance sport is also looked into because of its largely Euro-centric origin. This chapter then looks into the extent to which the concerned IF has been lax in implementing the WADA Code. The matter is analyzed on the basis of the empirical report generated on this issue by various researchers. The same is also done through the few cases that have been discussed and debated before CAS. This chapter argues that the implementation of the WADA Code within a small federation is a feasible proposition if the members are not struggling for funds and there are no other structural constraints. Importantly, the recognition process of smaller IFs should ensure that there is effective compliance with the WADA Code. Being a relatively older Non-Olympic sport, Dance sport should develop a robust compliance mechanism. Both World Anti-Doping Agency (WADA) and IOC should test the compliance level when they review the recognition granted to such sports. Importantly, such testing needs to be done more stringently when the sport is proposed to be included in the Olympic program.

Chapter 6 evaluates the compliance enforcement within the Non-Olympic sport. The issue of Non-Olympic sport failing in their Code compliance measures is not disputed, though the non-compliance with World Anti-Doping Agency (WADA) Code is not unique or confined to the Non-Olympic sports. However, their amenability to the jurisdiction of WADA depends upon their zeal to be part of the Olympic program. If the Non-Olympic sports are content to be recognized by the International Olympic Committee (IOC) then one cannot argue that they will be Code compliant. For their target of being recognized by IOC is fulfilled. They have nothing much to achieve. The popularity of the sport within the domestic market will also determine the extent of compliance. If the sport is popular within the domestic market, then there is no incentive for the Non-Olympic sport to undertake additional burden vis-à-vis Code compliance. Consequently, the relevance of any measure of compliance is effective if it is directly connected with the Olympics and its associated activities. Thus, for a Non-Olympic sport to comply with the WADA Code is purely a voluntary act. Hence, it is the responsibility of the WADA and the IOC to ensure that the level of compliance within the Non-Olympic sport is similar to the level within the Olympic sport, which has to be done by being proactive vis-à-vis the Non-Olympic sport. This chapter, therefore, looks into the roles and responsibilities of the WADA and IOC vis-à-vis sports in general. This chapter begins by analyzing the Code monitoring responsibilities of the various stake holders, primarily, the WADA and IOC. It looks into the standards developed for determining compliance failure and International standards that are in place vis-à-vis compliance measures of the various stake holders. It primarily focuses on the consequence for the IFs for non-compliance. This chapter then looks into the compliance enforcement efforts with respect to the Non-Olympic sports. The role of WADA and IOC is especially looked into to understand the importance of the Non-Olympic sport within the framework of anti-doping regulation. This chapter also tries to investigate the rationale behind extending the Code compliance responsibilities to the State signatories. This chapter questions the rationale of bringing the State into the picture and argues that insofar as the Non-Olympic sports are concerned, the State ought not to be held liable. The process of recognition and de-recognition is exclusively the domain of IOC; hence, States cannot be blamed for their laxities. This holds true even more for those Non-Olympic sports that do not depend on State funding. Hence, the WADA Code compliance cannot be used by IOC to usurp the sovereignty of the State. An exception ought to be made in case of Non-Olympic sports in this regard.

Objectives

This book aims to make the reader aware of the following:

1.   The concept of Non-Olympic sports and its difference from Olympic sports
2.   The doping problem within Non-Olympic sports

3. The extent of implementation of WADA within the selected Non-Olympic sports
4. The extent of a conflict between State sovereignty and IOC-WADA hegemony.

2 Non-Olympic Sports and Wada Code—The Twain Needs to Meet

Introduction

The recognition of a sport by the International Olympic Committee (herein-after IOC) is pre-conditioned upon, among others, the WADA Code compliance. The question, however, is: how is the WADA Code compliance to be judged? Further, recognition does not mean that the sport will automatically be part of the grand spectacle called the Olympic Games. The recognition of an International Federation, however, is the first step toward getting admitted to the hallowed halls of the Olympics. The sport gets the chance to be called an Olympic sport. The athletes/players get the chance to win Olympic medals and bask in the Olympic glory. The Olympic Charter is the document that lays down the foundation for such recognition by the IOC. Unfortunately, the Charter is completely silent as to the process of granting such recognition. The only thing that appears to be clear is the fact that the ultimate arbiter of such a decision is the IOC. The dominance of IOC means that the designation of activity as a sporting activity is ambiguous. It depends on the whims and fancies of the IOC. Interestingly, the criteria for recognition of a sport are, however, the same across the board. The uniform standard appears equitable but it creates problems at two levels. At the level of compliance postrecognition, there is a clear disparity between the Olympic sports and the Non-Olympic sports. The sports persons are subjected to different standards of scrutiny and regulations depending upon the level of performance. The sports persons/athletes participating in the Olympics are required to undergo rigorous tests, as part of the WADA Code compliance. The athletes/sports persons, as part of the Olympic sports, are constantly under the spotlight. Hence their actions are regularly scrutinized for determining rule violations. On the other hand, Non-Olympic sports persons/athletes fall under the radar. The level of scrutiny that they are subjected to is minimal. They neither have to bear the rigors of the system nor are they living under the fear of constant threat to career and livelihood. The present system creates two different worlds within sports. It dilutes the importance of the WADA Code since Non-Olympic sports are granted recognition by satisfying only the formal criteria. There is no compulsion or process that ensures substantive compliances. This chapter questions the very model

DOI: 10.4324/9781003082309-2

adopted by the IOC to grant recognition. It questions the rationale of insisting on WADA compliance. It begins by analyzing and surveying the Olympic system and highlights the various processes that are involved before a sport gains recognition by IOC. It looks into the consequence of being an IOC-recognized sport. Next, this chapter looks into the role of WADA in the entire process of recognition. It analyzes the WADA Code (both 2015 and 2021) to understand as well as explain the impact of the Code on the process of recognition. It compares the compliance level of the Non-Olympic sport with the Olympic sport. This chapter concludes by arguing that WADA Code compliance need not be the pre-condition for grant of recognition to a sport.

Olympic System and Sports' Recognition—A Puzzling Process

The Olympic System is defined and designed by the Olympic Charter, which proclaims itself as the Constitution of the sporting world.[1] The Olympic system comprises primarily the IOC, the International Federations (IFs), and the National Olympic Committees (NOCs).[2] The Organizing Committees of the Olympic Games are also co-opted as an integral part of this system. This set up, however, does not appear to have space for the athletes.[3] Hence, in the case of recognition of new sports, the entire negotiation appears to be confined at an administrative level. The supremacy of the IOC in granting recognition to IFs/events is codified in the Charter. Rule 2's Bye-Law and Rule 3 detail out just one criterion for getting recognized by the IOC. The same, as mentioned earlier, is the compliance with the Olympic Charter.[4] Thus, a review of the Olympic Charter is necessitated to identify the process of recognition. The Charter is a holistic document that not only maps out the mission of the Olympic movement but also explains the IOC's Organizational structure.[5] As per the Charter, the entire process of recognition and de-recognition is controlled by the Session. The Session is the highest decision-making body of the IOC.[6]

As per Rule 18, subrule 2, clause 2.8, the Session has the power "to decide on the awarding or withdrawal by the IOC of full recognition to or from NOCs, associations of NOCs, IFs, associations of IFs and other organisations."[7] No other body within the IOC has similar powers. Rule 25 specifies the preconditions that are mandatory for the IF to get recognition from the Session.[8] Apart from complying with the Charter, compliance with the WADA Code is a sine qua non for all the IFs applying for recognition. Rule 25 declares that WADA Code needs to be mandatorily adopted and implemented by the IFs. Another document that needs to be complied with mandatorily is the Olympic Movement Code on the Prevention of Manipulation of Competitions.[9] Rule 40 is another provision within the Charter, which specifies the condition for participation in the Olympic Games.[10] Herein too, mandatory compliance with WADA Code is required. The caveat though is that unlike Rule 25, Rule 40 presupposes that the sports are recognized. Hence, the scope of Rule 40 is confined to the determination of eligibility of a competitor, team official, or other team personnel. Finally, we have Rule 43 emphatically declaring that "Compliance with the World Anti-Doping Code and the Olympic Movement Code on the Prevention of Manipulation of Competitions is mandatory for the whole Olympic Movement."[11] Insofar as inclusion or exclusion from an edition of the Olympic Games is concerned, the same is determined in accordance with Rule 45.

The recognition of a sport by the IOC does not guarantee automatic inclusion in the Olympic Games. The Rule 45 subrule 2.1 states that the sports program "includes all sports for a specific edition of the Olympic Games, as determined by the Session from among the sports governed by the IFs recognised by the IOC ('the sports programme')."[12] Thus, the sports/IF may be IOC recognized but inclusion in the Olympic Games is decided by the Session. The IF itself has no role to play there. The Charter does spell out the "Mission and role of the IFs within the Olympic Movement" in Rule 26.[13] However, the same places the IFs only in the supporting role.[14] The predominant role of the IF is to take all measures necessary to support the IOC, promote the Olympic Movement, and participate in all IOC-mandated activities.[15] Furthermore, the IF has the responsibility to enforce the technical aspects of its sports in Olympic Games.[16] The same, however, is to be done in keeping with the mandate of the Olympic Charter. This being the status of the Ifs, it is obvious that their role in getting recognition for their sports is limited. The dominance of the IOC in determining the status of a sport is unequivocally established through the Charter.

Against this background, the process an IF needs to follow to claim recognition from the IOC is ambiguous. The IOC Charter does not lay down any guidelines in this regard. The Charter is all about IOC, the Olympic Games, and the Olympic Movement. Hence, if a sport has to hope to gain legitimacy within the Olympics, it has to rely on the whims and fancies of the IOC. One can though draw certain conclusions from the reading of the Olympic Charter, viz.,

a)   The sport needs to have codified rules before it can apply for recognition by the IOC.
b)   The said sport has to have a governing body with a defined hierarchy within.
c)   The said sport has to have a clean record in terms of match manipulation and doping.
d)   The said sport has to strictly comply with the mandate of the IOC Charter.
e)   The said sport has to strictly comply with the WADA Code.[17]

The catch is that these aforementioned requirements do not guarantee that the sport will be recognized by the IOC. Thus, there is a glaring gap between the reality and the theory pertaining to the recognition of a sport. It is important to further understand that even if a sport gets lucky enough to be recognized by the IOC, it will continue to be regarded as Non-Olympic sports. For the journey from becoming a recognized sport to an Olympic sport is long and uncertain. And it is this uncertainty that haunts Non-Olympic sports. For they continue with their efforts at graduating to Olympic sport.

From Sport to Non-Olympic Sport—Tracing the Journey

Non-Olympic sports first and foremost struggle to get recognition as sports. Sports, as we understand, is distinguishable from play or activity for amusement. An activity indulged for amusement and recreation is not ruled by structures. It is an informal set of activities that one indulges in for leisure.[18] On the contrary, sports that vie for a place within the Olympic pantheon are codified, have organized structures, maintain records of performances, have inbuilt procedure dispensing reward and punishment, and are commercialized.[19] The commercialization also ensures that they are competitive and generate suspense and thrill to keep the fans glued. The support from fans is a key to gauging the popularity of a sport.[20] And, the popularity of a sport is a key element in helping the sport to campaign for recognition by the IOC. As mentioned earlier, it is this recognition by the IOC that converts a sport into a Non-Olympic sport. The consistency of events held and tournaments conducted also adds stability to a sport. This enhances the chances of the sport to be considered as a candidate fit for recognition by the IOC.[21] There is a pertinent question that one needs to answer before proceeding viz., what are the perks of being recognized by the IOC?

There is a detailed organizational structure that the Non-Olympic sport currently has. A detailed study of this organizational maze is necessary to understand the perks of being a Non-Olympic sport. The ASSOCIATION OF IOC RECOGNISED INTERNATIONAL SPORTS FEDERATIONS (ARISF) is the body comprising the Non-Olympic sport.[22] This is the only body recognized by the IOC, which is authorized to represent the interests of Non-Olympic sports.[23] As indicated earlier, the IOC Charter provides basic guidelines for a sport to be recognized as a Non-Olympic sport. As soon as a sport is recognized as a Non-Olympic sport, they become eligible to be members of the ARISF.[24] The process of gaining membership in the ARISF is pretty simple and straightforward. The only criteria for getting the membership of the ARISF is to be recognized by the IOC. The converse is thus true that the membership is lost the moment the IOC withdraws its recognition. The membership is also lost upon the concerned sports getting the status of an Olympic sport. Article 7 of the "Statutes" of the ARISF details the procedure of gaining membership to the association.[25]

The Non-Olympic sport, upon gaining the IOC recognition, has to apply in writing for the membership of the ARISF. The President of the ARISF then vets the claims made in the said application. In effect, the only point which the President of the ARISF needs to look into is to test the veracity of the claim. Thus, the vetting process essentially is all about confirming the "recognition status by the IOC."[26] The president, however, is not authorized to approve the inclusion formally. The power to formally approve the inclusion of new members to ARISF is with the General Assembly.[27] The General Assembly is the highest decision-making body of the ARISF. As per Article 10 of the ARISF Statutes, the General Assembly is empowered to

1. bring in changes within the Statutes,
2. elect office bearers including the president and vice-president of the ARISF,
3. formally approve Annual Statement of Accounts,
4. relieve the office bearers from their designated responsibilities,
5. decide upon and formally approve the requisite membership fees,
6. formally approve the inclusion of new members to ARISF,
7. remove members from ARISF, and
8. formally notify the dissolution of the ARISF.[28]

In addition to all the above, the General Assembly has residuary powers to decide upon all other matters as covered by the ARISF Statutes.[29]

Inclusion of the Non-Olympic sport within the ARISF is exceedingly beneficial to the concerned sports. It provides them with a platform for canvassing their case of being granted the status of an Olympic sport.[30] This was indeed the idea that incentivized the IFs of the Non-Olympic sport to join hands and found ARISF in the year 1984.[31] The ARISF statutes through Article 5 spell out the objective of ARISF.[32] A review of the same firmly establishes that ARISF exists to help its members secure a place in the Olympic program. And the same is sought to be achieved by promoting the Olympic ideals. Accordingly, Article 5 states that ARISF has the following objectives:

1. To discuss all matters pertaining to Olympism and the Olympic movement as well as the role to be played by the recognized IFs within the Olympic system.
2. To uphold the interests common to all its members in order to facilitate better coordination and promotion of Olympic ideals.
3. To ensure cooperation among the members as well as with the non-members.
4. To effectively represent its members in all matters pertaining to Olympic Charter, the Olympic Congress, Olympic Solidarity, the Olympic Games, and the Olympic Movement.
5. To ensure that both ARISF and its members can harmoniously co-exist.
6. To nominate its members to various International Sports Organisations.
7. To widely participate in the IOC Programs, projects, and the IOC Congress.
8. To promote solidarity and friendship as well as cooperation among the members.
9. To facilitate the inclusion of its members in the Olympic program.[33]

ARISF's Statutes thus appear to be a B-grade version of the Olympic Charter. For its predominant objective appears to promote the ideals of the Olympic Charter. Article 8 clause 2 declares that

> The fundamental principles of the Olympic Charter shall prevail in all actions taken by ARISF and its Members. Rules and regulations, if issued by ARISF, shall not conflict with or derogate from those principles.[34]

Against such an environment, the Statutes understandably do not provide for any method of testing the compliances. The monitoring of the member's compliance with the Olympic Charter appears to be left to the IOC. This is clear from Article 7, which outlines the eligibility criteria for gaining membership in ARISF.[35] As mentioned earlier, recognition by the IOC is the only eligibility criterion for such a membership. Consequently, the obligation undertaken by ARISF is limited and that also has a bearing on the up-gradation of a Non-Olympic sport. Since the Non-Olympic sport has to only satisfy the IOC, compliance is the individual responsibility of the IF of such sport. Understandably, then the Statutes of ARISF are confined to only propagating the interests of its members. The presumption in favor of its members being compliant with the IOC Charter is beyond any contest. This assumption equally applies to compliance with WADA Code. And, in the absence of any mechanism to test the actual compliances, the IFs are absolutely on their own.

The lax approach toward compliances with the WADA Code and other mandates of the IOC Charter is, however, the norm. An IF eligible to be a member of ARISF is all set to become part of the larger Olympic structure. Hence, it is not in the interest of Non-Olympic sports to demand stringent regulation vis-à-vis compliances. Once a Non-Olympic sport becomes a member of ARISF, it automatically becomes a member of the Global Association of International Sports Federations (GAISF).[36] GAISF is one of the five recognized associations of IFs under the umbrella of the IOC.[37] A look at the other associations in this list will establish the intricate connection between ARISF and IOC. The IOC-recognized IF associations, apart from ARISF and GAISF, are the Association of Summer Olympic International Federations (ASOIF), Association of the International Olympic Winter Sports Federations (AIOWF), and Alliance of Independent Recognized Members of Sport (AIMS).[38] Of these, the ASOIF and AIOWF are associations of Olympic sports unlike the other three. We have noted earlier that ARISF is the association of Non-Olympic sports. In contrast, AIMS is the association of IFs that are not recognized by the IOC. An IF, being a member of AIMS though, can strive and gain recognition as Non-Olympic sports.[39]

One can draw a pattern from the above discussion as to the process which will help a sport gain the status of a Non-Olympic sport. First and foremost the pre-requisites of sport, as noted earlier, need to be established. Once the said point is taken care of, then the IF has the option of becoming a member of AIMS. Since the membership to AIMS is based on non-IOC-recognized sports, any sport can be a member of AIMS. And since AIMS is recognized by IOC, it provides a platform to the members of canvassing for recognition by the IOC. Once a sport, via AIMS, is successful in getting IOC recognition, they graduate to the status of Non-Olympic sports. And once declared a Non-Olympic sport, the eligibility to be a member of ARISF is gained. And once ARISF admits such a Non-Olympic sport within its fold, the process is complete. The next struggle is for the Non-Olympic sport to gain admission within the Olympic program and become an Olympic sport. The problem, however, is at the stage where a sport is recognized as a Non-Olympic sport. For it is at this stage that the laxity in compliance with the WADA Code creates an inherent disparity among the sports. The laxity in compliance with WADA Code thus leads to a more favorable treatment for Non-Olympic sports vis-à-vis Olympic sports. And the same also challenges the effectiveness of the WADA Code.

WADA Code 2015 and Non-Olympic Sports—Upping the Ante?

The 2015 Code revision was in response to the earlier criticism of the WADA Code.[40] Hence, the compliance standards were more stringent and the objective was to increase vigilance. The same, however, did not prevent the sporting scandals as is evident from the Russian doping scandal.[41] In the light of the Russian doping scandal, the 2015 Code underwent further revisions and various provisions were re-looked into.[42] Given this background, the requirement of compliances by Non-Olympic sport needs to be understood. One further needs to assess the reach of WADA vis-à-vis the Non-Olympic sports. One also needs to look into the checks and balance that exists to test the compliance level of the Non-Olympic sports. Thus, one needs to survey the provisions within the WADA Code, which are mandatory for anti-doping regulations. The current version that is in force is the 2021 WADA Code.[43] A comparison of the 2015 version with the 2021 version of the Code will help us in understanding the compliance requirements. This understanding is necessary to outline the compliance burden on Olympic sports. Importantly, it will help contrast the inherent disparity in compliance requirement between the Olympic sports and the Non-Olympic sports.

The 2015 Code was amended in 2017[44] as well as 2019[45] to close the loopholes identified in the light of the Russian doping scandal.[46] However, this was not thought to be good enough to check anti-doping violations. Hence, the 2021 Code was finalized and brought into force. The 2015 Code though did improve upon the 2009 version in its stringency.[47] A comparison of the two versions reveals the salient features of the 2015 Code. To start, the 2015 Code increased the sanction period from 2 years to 4 years.[48] Further, the Articles on violations were expanded to declare more infringements as amounting to anti-doping rule violations.[49] Another important aspect of the 2015 Code has been to incorporate and highlight the role of investigations and intelligence gathering. Investigations and intelligence gathering has been included in the 2015 Code as an important tool to check anti-doping rule violations.[50] The 2015 Code has also increased the limitation period to 10 years from the erstwhile 8 years. This extension is closely connected with the importance given to investigations and intelligence gathering. For such investigation and intelligence, data will take a while to reveal sophisticated anti-doping rule violations.[51]

The 2015 Code has also been expanded to cover the actions of Athlete support personnel. Hence, the use of prohibited methods and substance by the athlete support personnel will attract disciplinary action.[52] The 2015 Code thus enhances the role and responsibility of the athlete as well as its team. Importantly, the 2015 Code has eliminated any possibility of challenging the WADA-approved testing methods.[53] These methods are presumed to be valid and in case of any challenges to be made, WADA has to be notified first. The notice to WADA is a mandatory requirement for the athletes. WADA has to be informed about the basis of such challenge, and on its request, CAS shall constitute a panel of scientific experts. This panel is to assist CAS in determining the validity of the challenge.[54] Thus, the rigor of the 2015 Code makes it difficult for the athlete to fight the anti-doping system established by WADA. This rigor was further enhanced on November 15, 2017,[55] through amendments pertaining to the incorporation of the International Standard of Code Compliance by Signatories (ISCCS). This amendment was brought into effect on April 1, 2018.[56]

The ISCCS elaborates upon the roles and responsibilities of the signatories in order to comply with the standards laid down therein. Accordingly, the Articles of the Code were amended to enable the signatories to implement ISCCS.[57] Further, the amendments as well as the ISCCS elaborate upon the consequence that the signatories will face in the case of compliance failure.[58] Though ISCCS is mandatory for the signatories, its impact on Non-Olympic sport has been negligible. The same is evident from the nature of challenges brought before CAS, post these amendments. Another amendment was introduced on May 16, 2019, and brought into effect on June 1, 2019. The amendment was introduced to Article 7.4 requiring the laboratories to report atypical findings.[59] Thus, the amendments to the 2015 Code had only upped the ante for the athletes participating in Olympic sports. In such a scenario, the athletes participating in Olympic sports have no option but to abide by the system. CAS decisions post-2015 Code show the extent of the challenge faced by the Olympic sports' athlete within WADA. These decisions also reveal the kind of life a Non-Olympic sports' athlete has. For the Non-Olympic sports' athlete is not caught within the excruciating burden of proof that WADA imposes. Importantly, there appears to be a lack of scrutiny within the Non-Olympic sports vis-à-vis WADA compliance.

This lack of scrutiny is evident from the fact that between 2015 and 2020, hardly four to five cases of doping, within the Non-Olympic sports, have been arbitrated by CAS. This is evident from the CAS database.[60] A glance through the WADA website too paints the same picture.[61] This cannot lead to a conclusion that the 42 members of the ARISF have been less truant than their

Olympic counterparts. On the contrary, this proves the presence of a gaping hole in reporting of anti-doping violations by Non-Olympic sports. And the same challenges the efficacy of the WADA Code. Such a lack of scrutiny is problematic due to the severity of the consequences of anti-doping violations. In *F. v. Athletics Kenya (AK)*,[62] CAS declared that it is the duty of an experienced international athlete to take all precautions to avoid anti-doping rule violations (ADRV).[63] In this case, the ADRV was due to ingestion of a cough syrup containing a prohibited substance. The contention of the athlete that she trusted the pharmacist was rejected. CAS insisted that she ought to have consulted a doctor before consuming the cough syrup.[64] Thus, the athlete is burdened with a behavior not expected from a non-athlete, and there is no scope for letting the guards down. One can argue that the Non-Olympic sport, being a signatory of the WADA Code, is also subject to the same burden. However in reality, it is only the athletes participating in Olympic sports who appear to face the brunt.

The WADA Code imposes the responsibility of adopting, implementing, and enforcing anti-doping rules on the IFs. Hence, the IFs for Non-Olympic sport, like their counterpart in the Olympic sport, are autonomous in terms of compliance with the Code. However since strict WADA Code compliance is a mandatory condition to participate in the Olympics, there is no scope of laxity for the concerned IFs. The fallout from the Russian doping scandal is a clear example of the same.[65] As soon as it was established that Russia violated all the norms laid down in the WADA Code, widespread sanctions were imposed.[66] The sanctions affected the athletes to the extent that their chance of participating in the Olympics was ruled out.[67] The athletes were hauled up by both the IOC and WADA since they were amenable to the jurisdiction of both. Additionally, the IFs affected by the scandal too faced criticism and had to go for widespread reforms. The Russian scandal thus threatened to devalue and destabilize the entire anti-doping system.[68] The backlash was so severe because the main affected entities were Olympic sports. None of the 42 members of the ARISF has been ever involved in a scandal of such magnitude. This is so because Non-Olympic sports are not under the same level of scrutiny as Olympic sports. A review of the 2021 Code too reveals the extent of disparity between the Olympic sports and the Non-Olympic sports.

2021 Code and Non-Olympic sports—An Ambiguous Narrative

The 2021 Code has come into force since January 1, 2021, and is dictating the ongoing anti-doping narrative.[69] This narrative is based on ideals similar to those in the older versions of the Code. To start, it is declared that the purpose of the 2021 Code is to protect the athlete's right to participate in doing free sport. The same is achieved through the promotion of athlete's "health, fairness, and equality."[70] In addition, effective implementation of the WADA Code across the world is sought to be achieved among others through Rule of law. The same includes efforts on the part of WADA

> to ensure that all relevant stakeholders have agreed to submit to the Code and the International Standards, and that all measures taken in application of their anti-doping programs respect the Code, the International Standards, and the principles of proportionality and human rights.[71]

As per this statement, the WADA has the duty to ensure that all signatories, including the Non-Olympic sports, strictly comply with the Code. As was explained earlier, in practice though, WADA's effective monitoring appears to be confined to the Olympic sports. Nonetheless, on paper the Code, under its various provisions, outlines the role of WADA, in ensuring compliance across the board. To begin with, WADA has imposed the responsibility "for conducting all aspects of Doping Control"[72] on the individual anti-doping organizations.

These organizations include IOC, IFs, and other sports organizations that are signatories to the WADA Code. Thus, WADA is to act as a watchdog to ensure that there are no deviations from the Code provisions. In addition, it is the responsibility of individual athlete and athlete support personnel to know "what constitutes an anti-doping rule violation and the substances and methods which have been included on the Prohibited List."[73] Herein again WADA has delegated the responsibility of compliance and retained the supervisory role. And of all the stakeholders in the anti-doping system, the athletes have the greatest burden. For Article 2.1.1 insists that

> It is the Athletes' personal duty to ensure that no Prohibited Substance enters their bodies. Athletes are responsible for any Prohibited Substance or its Metabolites or Markers found to be present in their Samples. Accordingly, it is not necessary that intent, Fault, Negligence or knowing Use on the Athlete's part be demonstrated in order to establish an anti-doping rule violation.[74]

This Article thus incorporates the strict liability principle that is at the heart of the WADA-designed anti-doping program. This principle has been upheld through various CAS decisions as well as legal opinions. The same is regarded as a sine qua non for ensuring the efficacy of the WADA Code for, the burden is on the athlete and not on the anti-doping organizations.[75] The comment to Article 2.1.1 clarifies that "[a]n antidoping rule violation is committed under this Article without regard to an Athlete's Fault."[76] Further, the Code in the definition section at Appendix 1 defines strict liability as

> [t]he rule which provides that under Article 2.1 and Article 2.2, it is not necessary that intent, Fault, Negligence, or knowing Use on the Athlete's

part be demonstrated by the Anti-Doping Organization in order to establish an anti-doping rule violation.[77]

Thus, an athlete is proven to be guilty the moment ADRV is established. In such a scenario, lack of scrutiny vis-à-vis compliance on the part of the Non-Olympic sports is problematic. The lax attitude toward Non-Olympic sports automatically gives the concerned athlete an upper hand over the athletes from Olympic sports. And there are more than enough cases to document the devastating effect of the strict liability rule. In *USA Shooting & Q./Union Internationale de Tir (UIT)*,[78] it was held that "It is true that a strict liability test is likely in some sense to be unfair in an individual case."[79] However, the "requirement of intent would invite costly litigation that may well cripple federations—particularly those run on modest budgets—in their fight against doping."[80] And hence "in principle the high objectives and practical necessities of the fight against doping amply justify the application of a strict liability standard."[81]

And this justification has meant that till date, the athletes are doomed the moment an ADRV is established. Like its earlier version, the 2021 Code too has an elaborate list illustrating the varied scenario leading to ADRV. The list has been expanded to include newer instances of ADRV. To be specific, the 2021 Code has laid down the following 11 scenarios that amount to ADRV, viz.,

1. Presence of prohibited substance in the samples of the athlete (Article 2.1)
2. Use or attempted use of a prohibited substance or method (Article 2.2)
3. Refusal/Evasion/Failure to submit to sample collection (Article 2.3)
4. Whereabouts Failure (Article 2.4)
5. Tampering or attempted tampering with any part of the doping control (Article 2.5)
6. Possession of any of the prohibited substance or method (Article 2.6)
7. Trafficking or Attempted trafficking in prohibited substance or method (2.7)
8. Administration or attempted administration (either in-competition or out-of-competition) of prohibited substance or method
9. Complicity or attempted complicity in the form of assisting, encouraging, aiding, abetting, conspiring, covering up an ADRV, etc. (Article 2.9)
10. Prohibited Association
11. Acts amounting to discouragement from or retaliation for, reporting to authorities.[82]

Further, the 2021 Code incorporates the same standard of proof as in the older versions. Thus, an anti-doping organization has to establish an ADRV

to the comfortable satisfaction of the hearing panel, bearing in mind the seriousness of the allegation which is made. This standard of proof in all cases is greater than a mere balance of probability but less than proof beyond a reasonable doubt.[83]

On the other hand, the standard of proof vis-à-vis the athlete is a balance of probability.[84] Further like in the earlier versions, here too, the ADRV can be established through non-analytical methods. Thus, admissions of the athlete to ADRV, circumstantial evidence, third party account, or documentary evidence, etc., will all be relevant in establishing ADRV.[85] Continuity with earlier versions is equally maintained in the part dealing with the prohibited list. Thus, there will continue to be a yearly publication of the list. And, it will continue to have details of prohibited substances and methods.[86] Further, the list also indicates what are to be regarded as specified substance and specified methods. Importantly, the sole discretion of WADA in formulating the list is retained.[87] Consequently, there remains ambiguity as to the criteria for listing a substance/method as prohibited. The 2021 Code has for the first time recognized the larger public health concern relating to substance abuse. However, its effect in determining ADRV in the context of sports is awaited.[88] These additions, in expanding both the list of ADRV the prohibited list, do not change the ground realities vis-à-vis the Non-Olympic sports.

The Non-Olympic sports are supposed to adhere to the norms of establishing ADRV as well as the prohibited list. However, in the absence of any specific provisions pertaining to Non-Olympic sports or their process of recognition, things continue to be ambiguous. The same is the case with the provisions relating to Therapeutic Use Exemptions (TUEs).[89] These are mere replication of the earlier versions and hence do not help the Non-Olympic narrative. The other provisions relating to whereabouts information of athletes,[90] retired athletes returning to competition,[91] and investigations and intelligence gathering are also ambiguous.[92] In short, they do not address issues of accountability on the part of Non-Olympic sports. One can always argue that WADA Code applies across the board to all sports. However, the Olympic sports are by default caught in the WADA web due to their participation in the Olympics. Being Olympic sport means that they are constantly under the scrutiny of the anti-doping organizations. On the other hand, the Non-Olympic sports are comparatively low-key since absence from the Olympics means less publicity. There is also a lesser scope of backlash from the international community. Olympic sports are under pressure for they are expected to embody the ideals of the Olympic movement. These fundamental differences, therefore, make it essential that the WADA Code ought to have built-in systems that will ensure uniform compliance from all sports. Such a system is missing even within the provisions relating to the analysis of a sample that has been amended in the 2021 Code.

The changes introduced do expand the mandate of the anti-doping organization to continue with the testing of samples, without any limitation. However, as a safeguard, the consent of the Athlete is factored in. This aspect strengthens the ability of the anti-doping organization to continuously search for evidence of ADRV. However, it further weakens the position of the athlete and renders them more vulnerable. There is thus never-ending surveillance of the athletes through this continuous testing of samples.[93] Such an environment further highlights the problem of Non-Olympic sports having it easy when it comes to compliance issues. The 2021 Code though does authorize WADA

> in its sole discretion at any time, with or without prior notice [to] take physical possession of any Sample and related analytical data or information in the possession of a laboratory or Anti-Doping Organization. Upon request by WADA, the laboratory or Anti-Doping Organization in possession of the Sample or data shall immediately grant access to and enable WADA to take physical possession of the Sample or data.[94]

This provision being mandatory, non-cooperation with WADA will lead to ADRV. The obligation to cooperate is imposed on the signatories, viz., the anti-doping organizations. Logically, Non-Olympic sports automatically are covered by this provision. WADA thus has the opportunity to suo moto intervene in matters of non-compliance.

The comment to Article 6.8 states that WADA alone shall determine the grounds for such intervention. And the decision of WADA relating to the existence of "good cause" for such intervention is beyond any challenge.[95] However, only time will tell whether this power will be used by WADA to eliminate the existing discrepancy between Olympic sports and Non-Olympic sports. Since the sanction period for ADRV, subject to mitigating and other rules, is largely 4 years, such discrepancies are unfair.[96] Further, the defense of No Fault/Negligence[97] and the No Significant Fault/Negligence[98] has had a very low rate of success in the past. The scope of greater success under the new Code is awaited. Hence, the 2021 Code does not help matters much. Substantial relief can only be granted to all the athletes if at the ground level WADA can ensure effective compliance. And that, sadly, does not appear to have happened with the 2021 WADA Code. The 2021 Code does empower WADA to appeal to CAS without exhausting internal remedies.[99] In other words, if an anti-doping organization is lax in pursuing a case of ADRV, then WADA, subject to the determination of locus, can bypass the internal procedures and appeal directly to CAS. Thus, the 2021 Code has further enhanced the power of WADA to enable it to proactively enforce compliance with the Code. However, the ground-level realities as of now do not show any progress toward the same. It appears that the 2021 Code has not yet been able to narrow the chasm existing between Olympic sports and Non-Olympic sports. This is affirmed from Article 14.5, which elaborates upon the guidelines relating to "Doping Control Information Database and Monitoring of Compliance."[100]

The said Article puts the onus on the anti-doping organizations to report and submit details of compliances.[101] There is no responsibility imposed on WADA to ensure compliance. This, therefore, leads us back to the point from where we started. WADA's dependence on the anti-doping organizations is an example of a conflict of interest. For an anti-doping organization, violating the Code will not report correctly or give the true picture. Unless WADA independently monitors and investigates, there will not be any compulsion on the anti-doping organizations to be Code compliant. Interestingly in Article 20.7.14, WADA is empowered to "initiate its own investigations of anti-doping rule violations, non-compliance of Signatories and WADA-accredited laboratories, and other activities that may facilitate doping."[102] Interestingly, this is an elaboration of a similar provision under the 2015 Code.[103] Though till date, the evidence of a proactive investigation by WADA is yet to be witnessed in the field of the Non-Olympic sport. In the realm of Olympic sport though compliance is forced using the threat of bans. Article 20.1.6 clearly states that IOC has the responsibility to

> require all Athletes preparing for or participating in the Olympic Games, and all Athlete Support Personnel associated with such Athletes, to agree to and be bound by anti-doping rules in conformity with the Code as a condition of such participation or involvement.[104]

Consequently, non-compliance will inevitably lead to ban from the Olympics. And this threat of ban is more effective than any other to ensure the Olympic sports adhere to the WADA Code. The cases arising from the Russian doping scandal exemplify the drastic consequences for Olympic sports due to non-compliance with the Code.[105]

Code Conundrum for the Olympic Sports—Advantage Non-Olympic Sports!

Bye-Law 1.3 to Rule 45 of the Olympic Charter lists out the sports that are by default part of the Olympic Games.[106] A survey of the doping cases decided by CAS till date reveals that almost all of them, barring a few, relate to Olympic sports. These decisions also reveal the extent of scrutiny that the Olympic sports are under. In *World Anti-Doping Agency (WADA) v. Sri Lanka Anti-Doping Agency (SLADA) & Don Dinuda Dilshani Abeysekara,*[107] it was held that "[t]he need for an athlete to establish how a prohibited substance entered his or her system is a condition precedent to a finding of absence of fault or no significant fault." It was further reiterated that the "World Anti-Doping Code is intended to harmonise sanctions in such a way that is equally applicable to athletes young and old, amateur or professional."[108] Hence in this case, the fact that the athlete was a minor did not lead to any reduction in the sanction period.[109] In *Nikola Radjen v. Fédération Internationale de Natation (FINA),*[110] it was held that "Cheating is a key element of the notion of 'intent' as contained in the World Anti-Doping Code (WADA Code).[111] By using a Prohibited Substance, an athlete wishes to obtain an advantage in comparison to other athletes."[112] It was further stated that an

> athlete . . . who pleads for the application of No Significant Fault or Negligence . . . based on the fact that at the time he consumed the Prohibited Substance he was suffering from depressions, caused by his father's death,

has to provide . . . evidence of medical diagnosis for such disease, or testimony of an expert.[113]

Accordingly, CAS rejected the claim of the athlete that being in depression was the cause for the ADRV. CAS held that the athlete "knew that he used a Prohibited Substance and he did it deliberately."[114]

In *Niksa Dobud v. Fédération Internationale de Natation (FINA)*,[115] it was held that the proof of "[c]omfortable satisfaction is less than beyond reasonable doubt and more than on a balance of probabilities. The less probable the matter sought to be proved to that standard, the more cogent must be the evidence to prove it."[116] CAS further held that the "regulations governing test evasion do not require the governing body to establish why an athlete may have evaded a test; only that he had in fact done so."[117] Applying the said logic, CAS rejected the reasons given by the athlete for evading the tests. In doing so, CAS noted that "[t]he Panel is acutely conscious of the grave consequences to the Appellant of dismissal of the Appeal, especially in an Olympic year."[118] And this statement substantiates the arguments proffered herein. The consequence of missing the Olympics due to the ban is incomparable. Hence, the impact of the WADA Code on Olympic sports is most severe. Non-Olympic sports do not have the threat of losing out on the Olympics for there is no certainty about their inclusion in the Olympic program. And that is one of the key reasons for the Non-Olympic sports to be lax in terms of compliances. In *Nesta Carter v. International Olympic Committee (IOC)*,[119] the CAS declared that "[t]he possibility of the re-analysis of an athlete's sample within the applicable deadline of eight (8) years in the context of a global process of re-analysis of the samples collected at the Olympic Games can be exercised by the IOC."[120] According to CAS therefore except

> departures from clearly written international standards . . . which are stated within the rules to be fundamental . . . and subject to specific bias . . ., or bad faith or ill intentions and to any express provision to the contrary, there appears to be neither limitation nor reservation on the scope of the analysis.[121]

Hence, CAS declared that

> the re-analysis program is meant to protect the integrity of the competition results and the interests of athletes who participated without any prohibited substance and not the interests of athletes who were initially not detected for any reason and are later . . . found to have competed with a prohibited substance.[122]

This point is important for in-competition testing is only possible when the athlete participates in a competition. In the context of the Olympics, therefore, IOC has jurisdiction over athletes participating in the Olympic program.

Accordingly, IOC upon collecting samples also has the liberty to go for re-analyses. By default, therefore, Non-Olympic sports are saved from this level of scrutiny by virtue of their exclusion from the Olympic program. The Non-Olympic sports are accordingly less vulnerable to the diktats of WADA and IOC-run system. There is a lack of rigorous monitoring both at the pre-recognition stage and in the postrecognition stage for the Non-Olympic sports. In the above matter, CAS emphatically states that "[t]he Athlete knew or could have known that, as a participant at the Beijing [Olympic] Games, his samples could be retested at any time during the following eight years, and under any applicable method for any substance."[123] This level of pressure is not faced by Non-Olympic sports. For though the WADA Code is applicable to them, their systems are not proactive enough. Hence, the Non-Olympic sports' athletes are more privileged as compared to their Olympic sports' counterparts. The same is also evident from the statement of CAS where it reiterates that

> the rules applicable to each successive edition of the Olympic Games include a corresponding regulatory basis. These rules send a message to all participants at the Olympic Games, that they have the fundamental duty not to use any prohibited substance . . . .[124]

Hence if the athletes "fail to do so, they will not be entirely safe until the expiration of the statute of limitation, which was eight (8) years during the relevant period to this case, and has now been extended to ten (10) years."[125]

In *Ihab Abdelrahman v. Egyptian Anti-Doping Organization (EGY-NADO) & World Anti-Doping Agency (WADA) v. Ihab Abdelrahman & EGY-NADO,*[126] CAS underlined the relevance of the WADA Code by stating that

> while the relevant anti-doping rules are incorporated as the terms of the contractual relationship between an athlete and his or her international or national federation and/or the relevant anti-doping organisation, as the case may be, such anti-doping rules are incorporated in their entirety.[127]

Accordingly, like the Olympic sports, the Non-Olympic sports too have to follow the WADA Code in its entirety vis-à-vis their athletes. However in the absence of monitoring, as documented above, compliance is only formal but not substantive. In *World Anti-Doping Agency (WADA) v. Africa Zone V Regional Anti-Doping Organization & Anti-Doping Agency of Kenya (ADAK) & Athletics Kenya (AK) & Sharon Ndinda Muli,*[128] the stringency of the anti-doping system for Olympic sports is once again highlighted. Herein CAS declares that

> [i]n order to establish . . . how a prohibited substance entered an athlete's body, it is not sufficient for the athlete merely to protest their innocence . . . an athlete must adduce concrete evidence to demonstrate that a particular supplement, medication or other product that the athlete took contained the substance in question.[129]

And explaining the scope of the burden of proof on the athletes CAS reiterates that the "standard of proof of balance of probabilities requires an athlete to convince the CAS panel that the occurrence of the circumstances on which the athlete relies is more probable than their non-occurrence."[130] In accordance with this stance, CAS went on to reject the defense of the athlete against the finding of ADRV. As per CAS, the athlete "did not prove on the balance of probability how the prohibited substance entered her body or the origin of the prohibited substance."[131]

The quirky ways in which the athletes under the aegis of Olympic sports can get caught for ADRV are myriad. In *World Anti-Doping Agency (WADA) v. Gil Roberts*[132] is an example of such a scenario. Gil Roberts is "an American athlete specializing in the 200m and 400m sprint events, and a member of the gold medal 4x400m relay team during the 2016 Rio Olympic Games."[133] On March 24, 2017, the United States Anti-Doping Agency (USADA) conducted an out-of-competition test on the athlete. The sample tested positive for probenecid. The same is a "Specified Substance in the class of Diuretics and Masking Agents on the WADA List of Prohibited Substances."[134] Since ADRV was established, the burden shifted on the athlete to prove the source of the substance in his system. In the process of discharging this burden, the athlete pleaded No Fault or Negligence. As an arguendo, he pleaded No Significant Fault.[135] And this is where the athlete's argument became really interesting. In his defense, the athlete explained the circumstances under which the substance was likely to have been ingested. The athlete asserted that his girlfriend had sustained a sinus infection during her visit to India. As a consequence, she, with the help of her stepfather, bought an over-the-counter medicine. It was this medicine that contained, among others, probenecid. On the day of the out-of-competition test, his girlfriend took her usual dose of the medicine. Prior to undergoing the doping test, the athlete had kissed his girlfriend several times. In fact, he had kissed his girlfriend just before giving his sample for the doping test. Thus, the athlete firmly believed that it was the medicine that was the most probable source of probenecid. The athlete further added that he had no knowledge that his girlfriend was taking the medicine nor has he witnessed her taking the same.[136]

WADA challenged this argument of the athlete and countered the same by claiming it to be false concocted. As per WADA, the reasons for the athlete to present such a farfetched and concocted story "would be because, in fact, the probenecid had been taken by the Athlete as a masking agent to conceal the deliberate use of a performance enhancing substance."[137] However, CAS was convinced by the athlete's argument for the following reasons:

1. "To reject it requires the Panel to find in fact if not in strict law, that both the Athlete and more importantly, the other lay witnesses, conspired to mislead the Panel . . . the Panel would be presumptively reluctant to find that there was such a conspiracy."[138]

2. "The Panel had the opportunity to evaluate that testimony and the demeanor of the main witnesses, (athlete's girlfriend) and the Athlete, by sight and sound . . . the Panel judged them to be truthful, not least because they did not retreat from their evidence in any material way under sustained and powerful cross-examination."[139]

3. "The Panel . . ., however, note that (athlete's girlfriend), who had described her step-father as a film director, appeared wholly unaware of his actual occupation, which would be odd if they had pre-rehearsed an untruthful story."[140]

4. "If the Athlete was aware that he had taken some product which was or which contained a prohibited substance, the tests which he commissioned . . . [was] a wholly vain exercise . . . On the contrary, such behavior would only have been consistent with his genuine ignorance."[141]

5. The integrity of the Athlete's lawyer is impeccable irrespective of the fact that he has been "involved in a number of contamination cases (including two involving acts of kissing)."[142]

6. Athlete's girlfriend was genuinely unaware "that the Athlete's questions to her about whether and what she had recently consumed (and why indeed he was asking the questions at all) sprang from his lawyer's advice."[143]

7. WADA failed to explore or satisfactorily answer as to "Where did that capsule containing probenecid come from? How was it procured and by whom in such a short space of time?"[144]

8. The athlete would not have specifically procured a capsule "designed to acquit him, which itself served only to raise yet further questions as to what he was said to have innocently ingested."[145]

9. "The amount of probenecid found in the Athlete's out-of-competition sample would have no effect as a useful masking agent. Moreover, no plausible explanation for why probenecid would have been used by the Athlete was put forward by WADA."[146]

10. It was also noted that "the Athlete's biological passport was normal at all times and expressly did not raise any concerns or denote any suspicious activity."[147]

Based on these reasons, the Panel held that "it is more likely than not that the presence of probenecid in the Athlete's system resulted from kissing his girlfriend."[148]

In *World Anti-Doping Agency (WADA) v. South African Institute for Drug-Free Sport (SAIDS) & Gordon Gilbert*,[149] it was held, among other, that "[a]n athlete cannot simply plead his/her lack of intent without giving any convincing explanations to prove, by a balance of probability, that s/he did not engage in a conduct which s/he knew constituted an anti-doping rule violation . . . ."[150] It was further held that

A protestation of innocence, the lack of sporting incentive to dope, or mere speculation by an athlete as to what may have happened does not satisfy the required standard of proof (balance of probability) . . . unverified hypotheses are not sufficient.[151]

Accordingly, it was declared that "No reason of fairness is engaged with respect to an athlete found responsible for an intentional anti-doping rule violation."[152] In this the Sole Arbitrator, applying the principles relating to proof of lack of intent, found the athlete to be guilty of ADRV.[153] The defense of the athlete based on No Fault or Negligence and No-Significant Fault or Negligence was rejected. The Sole Arbitrator held that the athlete "has not proved that the anti-doping rule violation for which he is responsible was not intentional."[154] In *Fédération Internationale de Natation (FINA) v. Georgia Anti-Doping Agency (GADA) & Eastern Europe RADO & Irakli Bolkvadze*,[155] too it was held that "an athlete must adduce concrete evidence to demonstrate that the particular supplement etc. that s/he took contained the substance in question."[156] It was underlined by CAS that

> The WADA Code has been drafted to reflect the principle of proportionality, according to which there must be a balance between the relevance of the breach committed and the sanction imposed . . . the principle of proportionality is "built into" the WADA Code.[157]

Applying the principles as settled for establishing No Fault or Negligence and No Significant Fault or Negligence, the CAS held that "the Athlete did not prove on the balance of probability how the prohibited substance entered his body or the origin of the prohibited substance."[158] Thus, the stricture for the athletes under the aegis of Olympic sport continues to be in place without wavering. The decisions do not provide any escape route for these athletes. They continue to depend upon their luck and the CAS Panel hoping that the tide turns in their favor. However, the application of the mitigating circumstances appears to be an exception rather than the rule. Barring a one-off case, it is largely a scene loaded heavily against the athletes from the Olympic sports. In *Filip Radojevic v. Fédération Internationale de Natation (FINA)*,[159] for instance, CAS held that

> [t]he prescription of a medicinal product by an athlete's doctor does not excuse said athlete from investigating to their fullest extent that the medication at stake does not contain prohibited substances. Athletes cannot rely on the advice of their support personnel.[160]

Accordingly, it was reiterated that

> The concept of no significant fault or negligence requires more of an athlete than a conscious bona fide use of a prescribed medication. Athletes are required to seek information actively and to take precautions in order to avoid any ingestion of a prohibited substance.[161]

It was emphasized that "[a]n athlete must demonstrate the same level of diligence with regard to all substances included in the World Anti-Doping Agency Prohibited List irrespective of their capability of enhancing performances."[162]

CAS further pointed out that "[a]n athlete whose level of care and investigations was inexistent in relation to what should have been the perceived level of risk acts in a significantly negligent way."[163] CAS thus went on to hold that the athlete

> clearly has been completely passive and even careless with regard to his anti-doping duties. In addition to neglecting to check that the medicines prescribed [for] prohibited substances the Athlete failed to report the use of [such medicine] in the doping control form.[164]

CAS thus rejected the defense of the athlete based on No Significant Fault or Negligence. Similarly, in *World Anti-Doping Agency (WADA) v. Czech Anti-Doping Committee (CADC) & Czech Swimming Federation (CSF) & Kateřina Kašková,*[165] award of September 23, 2019, it was declared that the

> submissions, documents and evidence on behalf of the athlete must be persuasive that the occurrence of the circumstances which the athlete relies is more probable than their non-occurrence. It is not sufficient to suggest that the prohibited substance must have entered his/her body inadvertently from some supplements or other product.[166]

Accordingly CAS reiterated that the absence of

> proof of purchase, information as to the specific type of supplement used, by whom it is produced, etc. and absent any disclosure of the food supplement on the doping control form, there is no element substantiating the athlete's contention that s/he did use that product or that it was contaminated.[167]

Here too, the athlete failed to prove that the "violation was not intentional."[168] The cases relating to the Olympic sports thus highlight the problem of proving innocence under the WADA Code. And, the constant pressure that is there on the athletes trying their best to be on the right side of the WADA Code.

Conclusion

The Non-Olympic sport, with the doping cases score in single digit, needs to catch up with the Olympic sports in terms of compliance. And that can only be achieved if they seamlessly integrate within the compliance system of the WADA Code. However, the WADA Code has not incorporated any provision to ensure this integration. The role of ARISF is important in insisting on more rigorous monitoring of the compliance by the Non-Olympic sport. The ARISF needs to take a leaf out of the book of the Olympic sports. There has to be proper scrutiny before a sport is admitted as a member of the ARISF. Further, the ARISF should coordinate with the IOC to have proper screening before a sport is recognized. To insist on WADA Code compliance as a condition precedent to recognition of a sport by the IOC is problematic. This is so because such an insistence does not take into account the lack of monitoring to ensure actual compliance. In the absence of such monitoring, a sport just has to put in place formal compliance measures. IOC, without having any clear guidelines as to such monitoring, grants recognition based on the proof of formal compliance. Hence there is a failure of monitoring at the pre-recognition stage. As the caseload reveals even at the postrecognition stage, there are no strict compliances on the part of the Non-Olympic sport. Consequently, the insistence on WADA Code compliance by the IOC remains in letter but not in spirit. It becomes a mere paperwork without having any real-time impact on Non-Olympic sports. Further, such an insistence also has the potential of weakening the WADA Code and the entire anti-doping system. It also has the potential of increasing the burden on WADA to monitor sports at the pre-recognition stage. And a failure to do the same will undermine the legitimacy of WADA. Hence, it is advisable to do away with the requirement of WAD Code compliance. As the review in the next few chapters will reveal, the Non-Olympic sports might not be amenable to strict WADA Code compliance. Hence in the interest of all the stakeholders, it is important that the requirement of the WADA Code compliance be revisited. IOC needs to do the same to strengthen WADA as well as the anti-doping movement.

Notes

1. James B. Perrine, "Market Solutions to Olympic Problems: Do Athletes, Networks, and Sponsors Really Need the IOC?" *The University of New South Wales Law Journal*, vol. 22, 1999, p. 870
2. Olympic Charter, Rule 1-Composition and General Organization of the Olympic Movement (clause 2) [The Three Main Constituents of the Olympic Movement Are the International Olympic Committee ("IOC"), the International Sports Federations ("IFs") and the National Olympic Committees ("NOCs").]
3. Michael S. Straubel, "Doping Due Process: A Critique of the Doping Control Process in International Sport" *Dickinson Law Review*, vol. 106, 2001–2002, p. 523
4. Charter (n 2), Bye-law to Rule 2 [1. The IOC Executive Board may grant IOC patronage, upon such terms and conditions as it may consider appropriate, to international multisports competitions—regional, continental or worldwide—on condition that they take place in compliance with the Olympic Charter and are organised under the control of NOCs or associations recognised by the IOC, with the assistance of the IFs concerned and in conformity with their technical rules. 2. The IOC Executive Board may grant IOC patronage to other events, provided such events are in keeping with the goal of the Olympic Movement.]; Rule 3 Recognition by the IOC [1. The IOC may grant formal recognition to the constituents of the Olympic Movement. 2. The IOC may recognise as NOCs national sports organisations, the activities of which are linked to its mission and role. The IOC may also recognise associations of NOCs formed at continental or world level. All NOCs and

associations of NOCs shall have, where possible, the status of legal persons. They must comply with the Olympic Charter. Their statutes are subject to the approval of the IOC. 3. The IOC may recognise IFs and associations of IFs. 4. The recognition of associations of IFs or NOCs does not in any way affect the right of each IF and of each NOC to deal directly with the IOC, and vice-versa. 5. The IOC may recognise non-governmental organisations connected with sport, operating on an international level, the statutes and activities of which are in conformity with the Olympic Charter. In each case, the consequences of recognition are determined by the IOC Executive Board. 7. Recognition by the IOC may be provisional or full. Provisional recognition, or its withdrawal, is decided by the IOC Executive Board for a specific or an indefinite period. The IOC Executive Board may determine the conditions according to which provisional recognition may lapse. Full recognition, or its withdrawal, is decided by the Session. All details of recognition procedures are determined by the IOC Executive Board.]

5. Ibid [Introduction to the Olympic Charter-The Olympic Charter (OC) is the codification of the Fundamental Principles of Olympism, Rules and Bye-laws adopted by the International Olympic Committee (IOC). It governs the organisation, action and operation of the Olympic Movement and sets forth the conditions for the celebration of the Olympic Games. In essence, the Olympic Charter serves three main purposes: a) The Olympic Charter, as a basic instrument of a constitutional nature, sets forth and recalls the Fundamental Principles and essential values of Olympism. b) The Olympic Charter also serves as statutes for the International Olympic Committee. c) In addition, the Olympic Charter defines the main reciprocal rights and obligations of the three main constituents of the Olympic Movement, namely the International Olympic Committee, the International Federations and the National Olympic Committees, as well as the Organising Committees for the Olympic Games, all of which are required to comply with the Olympic Charter.]

6. Charter (n 2), Rule 17 Organisation [The powers of the IOC are exercised by its organs, namely: 1. the Session, 2. the IOC Executive Board, 3. the President.]

7. Ibid

8. Ibid Rule 25 Recognition of IFs [In order to develop and promote the Olympic Movement, the IOC may recognise as IFs international non-governmental organisations governing one or several sports at the world level, which extends by reference to those organisations recognised by the IFs as governing such sports at the national level. The statutes, practice and activities of the IFs within the Olympic Movement must be in conformity with the Olympic Charter, including the adoption and implementation of the World Anti-Doping Code as well as the Olympic Movement Code on the Prevention of Manipulation of Competitions. Subject to the foregoing, each IF maintains its independence and autonomy in the governance of its sport.]

9. Ibid

10. Ibid Rule 40 Participation in the Olympic Games* [To participate in the Olympic Games, a competitor, team official or other team personnel must respect and comply with the Olympic Charter and World Anti-Doping Code, including the conditions of participation established by the IOC, as well as with the rules of the relevant IF as approved by the IOC, and the competitor, team official or other team personnel must be entered by his NOC.]

11. Ibid

12. Ibid

13. Ibid Rule 26 Mission and role of the IFs within the Olympic Movement [1. The mission and role of the IFs within the Olympic Movement are: 1.1 to establish and enforce, in accordance with the Olympic spirit, the rule concerning the practice of their respective sports and to ensure their application; 1.2 to ensure the development

of their sports throughout the world; 1.3 to contribute to the achievement of the goals set out in the Olympic Charter, in particular by way of the spread of Olympism and Olympic education; 1.4 to support the IOC in the review of candidatures for organising the Olympic Games for their respective sports; 1.5 to assume the responsibility for the control and direction of their sports at the Olympic Games; 1.6 for other international multisport competitions held under the patronage of the IOC, IFs can assume or delegate responsibility for the control and direction of their sports; 1.7 to provide technical assistance in the practical implementation of the Olympic Solidarity programmes; 1.8 to encourage and support measures relating to the medical care and health of athletes. 2. In addition, the IFs have the right to: 2.1 formulate proposals addressed to the IOC concerning the Olympic Charter and the Olympic Movement; 2.2 collaborate in the preparation of Olympic Congresses; 2.3 participate, on request from the IOC, in the activities of the IOC commissions.]

14. Ibid
15. Ibid
16. Ibid
17. See generally Graham Scambler, "Sociology, Sport and Change: 1-Ancient to Modern" www.grahamscambler.com/sociology-sport-and-change-1-ancient-to-modern/ (accessed 10th January 2021)
18. James H. Frey and D. Stanley Eitzen, "Sport and Society" *The Annual Review of Sociology*, vol. 17, 1991, pp. 503–522
19. Stefan Szymanski, "A Theory of the Evolution of Modern Sport" *Journal of Sport History*, vol. 35, no. 1, 2008, pp. 1–32. JSTOR www.jstor.org/stable/26404949 (accessed 2nd February 2021)
20. Paavo Seppänen, "The Idealistic and Factual Role of Sport in International Understanding" *Current Research on Peace and Violence: Sports Relations & International Understanding*, vol. 5, no. 2–3, 1982, pp. 113–121. JSTOR www.jstor.org/stable/40724935 (accessed 2nd February 2021)
21. See generally Helen Jefferson Lenskyj, *Gender Politics and the Olympic Industry* (Palgrave Pivot, 2013)
22. Association of IOC Recognised International Sports Federations, "About Arisf-Who We Are" www.arisf.sport/who-we-are.aspx (accessed 13th January 2021)
23. International Olympic Committee, "Recognised Organisations" www.olympic.org/ioc-governance-affiliate-organisations (accessed 13th January 2021)
24. Association of IOC Recognised International Sports Federations (ARISF)-Statutes, Article 7-Membership [7.1 ARISF is composed of IFs that are recognised or provisionally recognised by the IOC according to Article 25 of the Olympic Charter as recognised IFs and whose sports are not full member of ASOIF or AIOWF. International Sports Federations that are not recognized by the IOC as recognised IFs cannot be a member of ARISF.] www.arisf.sport/download/arisf_statutes_as_adopted_at_ga_20170403_aarhus.pdf (accessed 21 February 2021)
25. (ARISF)-Statutes (n 24) Article 7—Membership [7.2 Each IF that is recognised or provisionally recognised by the IOC can affiliate as an ARISF member. IFs seeking ARISF membership must submit a written application to the ARISF President. The ARISF President shall confirm the membership request following verification of the recognition status by the IOC. 7.3 A Member will automatically lose its membership status when one or more of its disciplines are included as full member of ASOIF or AIOWF. A Member will also lose its membership should, for any reason whatsoever, the IOC decide to withdraw that member's recognition.]
26. Ibid
27. Ibid Article 10
28. Ibid Article 10.1 [The General Assembly is the highest authority of ARISF. It shall be held at least once a year and shall have all the powers in ARISF that, according

to governing law and these Statutes, have not been given to other bodies of ARISF. The General Assembly is empowered to: a) Approve and modify the Statutes b) Elect the President, the Vice-President, the Secretary General and the Council Members as well as the Financial Auditors. c) Approve the yearly statements of accounts. d) Discharge from responsibility the Council and the Financial Auditors. e) Determine the membership fees. f) Approve new Members. g) Exclude Members. h) Voluntarily dissolve ARISF. i) Decide on all other cases foreseen in these Statutes and the By-Laws

29. Ibid
30. Kurt Badenhausen, "How A Sport Becomes an Olympic Event" *Forbes* www. forbes.com/sites/kurtbadenhausen/2016/08/09/how-a-sport-becomes-an-olympic-event/?sh=295e5a3c2ce9 (accessed 13th February 2021)
31. (ARISF)-Statutes (n 24) Article 2 — Foundation and Duration [2.1 ARISF Was Founded in 1984 by the International Sports Federations (IFs) Recognised by the International Olympic Committee (IOC). 2.2 ARISF Is Established for an Indefinite Term.]
32. Ibid Article 5 — Objects
33. Ibid [The objectives of ARISF are: 5.1 To discuss matters raised by its members on questions of common interest, in relation to Olympism and the Olympic Movement and in relation to the role of recognised IFs as an integrated part of the Olympic Movement. 5.2 To coordinate and defend the common interests of its members in the above context. 5.3 To ensure close co-operation between its members, as well as other Sports Federations and organisations. 5.4 To act as a spokesman on behalf of its members in matters relating to the Olympic Charter, the Olympic Congress, Olympic Solidarity, the Olympic Games and the Olympic Movement in general. 5.5 To maintain the authority, independence and autonomy of its members and to ensure respect of the decisions made by the General Assembly. 5.6 To decide on nominations of ARISF representatives on International Sports Organisations To ensure the widest possible participation at IOC Congresses and in IOC Programs and Projects. 5.8 To encourage the convening of its members for the purpose of creating links of friendship, solidarity and collaboration between them. 5.9 To actively support the inclusion of the sports of its members in the Olympic Program. 5.10 Such other aims and objectives as may from time to time be defined by the General Assembly.]
34. Ibid Article 8—Independence and Autonomy of Member IFS
35. (ARISF)-Statutes (n 24), Article 7—Membership [7.1 ARISF is composed of IFs that are recognised or provisionally recognised by the IOC according to Article 25 of the Olympic Charter as recognised IFs and whose sports are not full member of ASOIF or AIOWF. International Sports Federations that are not recognized by the IOC as recognised IFs cannot be a member of ARISF. 7.2 Each IF that is recognised or provisionally recognised by the IOC can affiliate as an ARISF member. IFs seeking ARISF membership must submit a written application to the ARISF President. The ARISF President shall confirm the membership request following verification of the recognition status by the IOC. 7.3 A Member will automatically lose its membership status when one or more of its disciplines are included as full member of ASOIF or AIOWF. A Member will also lose its membership should, for any reason whatsoever, the IOC decide to withdraw that member's recognition.]
36. Global Association of International Sports Federations (GAISF), Members https://gaisf.sport/members/ (accessed 14th February 2021)
37. International Olympic Committee (n 23)
38. Ibid
39. "About AIMS" http://aimsisf.org/about-aims/ (accessed 14th February 2021)

40. "World Anti-Doping Code 2015 with 2019 Amendments" www.wada-ama.org/sites/default/files/resources/files/wada_anti-doping_code_2019_english_final_revised_v1_linked.pdf (accessed 1st February 2021)
41. Lovely Dasgupta, *The World Anti-Doping Code- Fit for Purpose?* (Routledge 2019)
42. Ibid
43. "World Anti-Doping Code 2021" www.wada-ama.org/sites/default/files/resources/files/2021_wada_code.pdf (accessed 1st February 2021)
44. Proposed Changes to Provisions in 2015 World Anti-Doping Code Relating to Compliance by Signatories, "2015 World Anti-Doping Code Amendments Adopted by Wada's Foundation Board on 16 November 2017 and to Come into Force on 1 April 2018" www.wada-ama.org/sites/default/files/2015_code_november2017_amendments_en.pdf (accessed 15th February 2021)
45. "Amendments to Article 7.4 of the Code Accepted by the World Anti-Doping Agency's Foundation Board on 16 May 2019 and to Come into Force on 1 June 2019" www.wada-ama.org/sites/default/files/resources/files/wada_article_7.4_modifications_en.pdf (accessed 15th February 2021)
46. Dasgupta (n 41)
47. "Significant Changes Between the 2009 Code and the 2015 Code, Version 4.0" www.wada-ama.org/sites/default/files/wadc-2015-draft-version-4.0-significant-changes-to-2009-en.pdf (accessed 15th February 2021)
48. Version 4.0 (n 47)
49. Ibid
50. Ibid
51. Ibid
52. Ibid
53. World Anti-Doping Code 2015 with 2019 Amendments, Article 3.2 Methods of Establishing Facts and Presumptions [Article 3.2.1 Analytical methods or decision limits approved by WADA after consultation within the relevant scientific community and which have been the subject of peer review are presumed to be scientifically valid. Any Athlete or other Person seeking to rebut this presumption of scientific validity shall, as a condition precedent to any such challenge, first notify WADA of the challenge and the basis of the challenge. CAS, on its own initiative, may also inform WADA of any such challenge. At WADA's request, the CAS panel shall appoint an appropriate scientific expert to assist the panel in its evaluation of the challenge. Within 10 days of WADA's receipt of such notice, and WADA's receipt of the CAS file, WADA shall also have the right to intervene as a party, appear amicus curiae or otherwise provide evidence in such proceeding.]
54. Version 4.0 (n 47)
55. Code (n 53) Article 12 Sanctions Against Signatories and Against Sporting Bodies that are not Signatories [12.1 The International Standard for Code Compliance by Signatories sets out when and how WADA may proceed against a Signatory for failure to comply with its obligations under the Code and/or the International Standards, and identifies the range of possible sanctions that may be imposed on the Signatory for such non-compliance. 12.2 Nothing in the Code or the International Standard for Code Compliance by Signatories restricts the ability of any Signatory or government to take action under its own rules to enforce the obligation on any other sporting body over which it has authority to comply with, implement, uphold and enforce the Code within that body's area of competence.]
56. "World Anti-Doping Code International Standard Code Compliance by Signatories April 2018" www.wada-ama.org/sites/default/files/resources/files/isccs_april_2018_0.pdf (accessed 15th February 2021)
57. Article 12 (n 55)

58. The current Standard in force is the World Anti-Doping Code International Standard for Code Compliance by Signatories 2021 [The following articles in the Code are directly relevant to the International Standard for Code Compliance by Signatories. They can be obtained by referring to the Code itself: • Article 12 Sanctions by Signatories Against Other Sporting Bodies • Article 13.6 Appeals from Decisions under Article 24.1 • Article 20 Additional Roles and Responsibilities of Signatories and WADA • Article 24 Monitoring and Enforcing Compliance with the Code and UNESCO Convention] www.wada-ama.org/sites/default/files/resources/files/international_standard_isccs_2020.pdf (accessed 15th February 2021)
59. Amendments to Article 7.4 (n 45)
60. Court of Arbitration for Sport, "Database" www.tas-cas.org/en/jurisprudence/archive.html (accessed 16th February 2021)
61. World Anti-Doping Agency, "Resources List" www.wada-ama.org/en/resources/search?f%5B0%5D=field_topic%3A138&f%5B1%5D=field_resource_type%3A125 (accessed 15th February 2021)
62. CAS 2015/A/3899
63. Ibid para 60
64. Ibid para 64
65. Dasgupta (n 41)
66. Ibid
67. Ibid
68. Ibid
69. "World Anti-Doping Code 2021" www.wada-ama.org/sites/default/files/resources/files/2021_wada_code.pdf (accessed 16th February 2021)
70. Ibid [The purposes of the World Anti-Doping Code and the World Anti-Doping Program which supports it are: •To protect the Athletes' fundamental right to participate in doping-free sport and thus promote health, fairness and equality for Athletes worldwide.]
71. Ibid
72. Code 2021 (n 69)
73. Ibid Article 2 [Anti-Doping Rule Violations]
74. Ibid
75. Dasgupta (n 41)
76. Code 2021 (n 69)
77. Ibid
78. CAS 94/129
79. Ibid para 14
80. Ibid para 15
81. CAS 94/129 (n 78) para 16
82. Code 2021 (n 69)
83. Ibid Article 3 Proof of Doping
84. Ibid
85. Ibid Article 3.2 [Methods of Establishing Facts and Presumptions Facts related to anti-doping rule violations may be established by any reliable means, including admissions.]
86. Ibid Article 4
87. Ibid [Article 4.3-Criteria for Including Substances and Methods on the Prohibited List WADA shall consider the following criteria in deciding whether to include a substance or method on the Prohibited List: 4.3.1 A substance or method shall be considered for inclusion on the Prohibited List if WADA, in its sole discretion, determines that the substance or method meets any two of the following three criteria: 4.3.1.1 Medical or other scientific evidence, pharmacological effect or experience that the substance or method, alone or in combination with other substances

or methods, has the potential to enhance or enhances sport performance; 4.3.1.2 Medical or other scientific evidence, pharmacological effect or experience that the Use of the substance or method represents an actual or potential health risk to the Athlete; 4.3.1.3 WADA's determination that the Use of the substance or method violates the spirit of sport described in the introduction to the Code. 4.3.2 A substance or method shall also be included on the Prohibited List if WADA determines there is medical or other scientific evidence, pharmacological effect or experience that the substance or method has the potential to mask the Use of other Prohibited Substances or Prohibited Methods. 4.3.3 WADA's determination of the Prohibited Substances and Prohibited Methods that will be included on the Pro-hibited List, the classification of substances into categories on the Prohibited List, the classification of a substance as prohibited at all times or In-Competition only, the classification of a substance or method as a Specified Substance, Specified Method or Substance of Abuse is final and shall not be subject to any challenge by an Athlete or other Person including, but not limited to, any challenge based on an argument that the substance or method was not a masking agent or did not have the potential to enhance performance, represent a health risk or violate the spirit of sport.]
88. Ibid
89. Ibid Article 4.4
90. Ibid Article 5.5
91. Ibid Article 5.6
92. Ibid Article 5.7
93. Ibid Article 6 [6.6 Further Analysis of a Sample After it has been Reported as Nega-tive or has Otherwise not Resulted in an Anti-Doping Rule Violation Charge After a laboratory has reported a Sample as negative, or the Sample has not otherwise resulted in an anti-doping rule violation charge, it may be stored and subjected to further analyses for the purpose of Article 6.2 at any time exclusively at the direc-tion of either the Anti-Doping Organization that initiated and directed Sample col-lection or WADA. Any other Anti-Doping Organization with authority to test the Athlete that wishes to conduct further analysis on a stored Sample may do so with the permission of the Anti-Doping Organization that initiated and directed Sample collection or WADA, and shall be responsible for any follow-up Results Manage-ment. Any Sample storage or further analysis initiated by WADA or another Anti-Doping Organization shall be at WADA's or that organization's expense. Further analysis of Samples shall conform with the requirements of the International Stand-ard for Laboratories.]
94. Code 2021 (n 69), Article 6.8
95. Ibid Comment to Article 6.8 [WADA would not, of course, unilaterally take pos-session of Samples or analytical data without good cause related to a potential anti-doping rule violation, non-compliance by a Signatory or doping activities by another Person. However, the decision as to whether good cause exists is for WADA to make in its discretion and shall not be subject to challenge. In particular, whether there is good cause or not shall not be a defense against an anti-doping rule violation or its Consequences.]
96. Code 2021 (n 69), Article 10
97. Ibid Article 10.5
98. Ibid Article 10.6
99. Ibid Article 13.1.3 [WADA Not Required to Exhaust Internal Remedies85 Where WADA has a right to appeal under Article 13 and no other party has appealed a final decision within the Anti-Doping Organization's process, WADA may appeal such decision directly to CAS without having to exhaust other remedies in the Anti-Doping Organization's process.]

100. Code 2021 (n 69), Article 14.5 [Doping Control Information Database and Monitoring of Compliance To enable WADA to perform its compliance monitoring role and to ensure the effective use of resources and sharing of applicable Doping Control information among Anti-Doping Organizations, WADA shall develop and manage a Doping Control information database, such as ADAMS, and Anti-Doping Organizations shall report to WADA through such database Doping Control-related information, including, in particular, a) Athlete Biological Passport data for International-Level Athletes and National-Level Athletes, b) Whereabouts information for Athletes including those in Registered Testing Pools, c) TUE decisions, and d) Results Management decisions, as required under the applicable International Standard(s). 14.5.1 To facilitate coordinated test distribution planning, avoid unnecessary duplication in Testing by various Anti-Doping Organizations, and to ensure that Athlete Biological Passport profiles are updated, each Anti-Doping Organization shall report all In-Competition and Out-of-Competition tests to WADA by entering the Doping Control forms into ADAMS in accordance with the requirements and timelines contained in the International Standard for Testing and Investigations. 14.5.2 To facilitate WADA's oversight and appeal rights for TUEs, each Anti-Doping Organization shall report all TUE applications, decisions and supporting documentation using ADAMS in accordance with the requirements and timelines contained in the International Standard for Therapeutic Use Exemptions. 14.5.3 To facilitate WADA's oversight and appeal rights for Results Management, Anti-Doping Organizations shall report the following information into ADAMS in accordance with the requirements and timelines outlined in the International Standard for Results Management: (a) notifications of anti-doping rule violations and related decisions for Adverse Analytical Findings; (b) notifications and related decisions for other anti-doping rule violations that are not Adverse Analytical Findings; (c) whereabouts failures; and (d) any decision imposing, lifting or reinstating a Provisional Suspension. 14.5.4 The information described in this Article will be made accessible, where appropriate and in accordance with the applicable rules, to the Athlete, the Athlete's National Anti-Doping Organization and International Federation, and any other Anti-Doping Organizations with Testing authority over the Athlete.]
101. Ibid
102. Code 2021 (n 69), Article 20.7- Roles and Responsibilities of WADA
103. CODE 2015 (n 40), Article 20.7.10 [To initiate its own investigations of anti-doping rule violations and other activities that may facilitate doping.]
104. Code 2021 (n 69)
105. Dasgupta (n 41)
106. Charter (n 2) [Bye-Law 1.3- The sports which may be included in the sports programme of the Games of the Olympiad are: 1.3.1 The sports, governed by the following IFs, which are currently included in the programme, namely:— International Association of Athletics Federations (IAAF);—World Rowing Federation (FISA);—Badminton World Federation (BWF);—International Basketball Federation (FIBA);—International Boxing Association (AIBA);— International Canoe Federation (ICF);—International Cycling Union (UCI); 83 Olympic Charter In force as from 17 July 2020—International Equestrian Federation (FEI);—International Fencing Federation (FIE);—International Association Football Federation (FIFA);—International Golf Federation (IGF);— International Gymnastics Federation (FIG);—International Weightlifting Federation (IWF);—International Handball Federation (IHF);—International Hockey Federation (FIH);—International Judo Federation (IJF);—United World Wrestling (UWW);—International Swimming Federation (FINA);—International Modern Pentathlon Union (UIPM);—World Rugby (WR);—World Taekwondo

Federation (WTF);—International Tennis Federation (ITF);—International Table
Tennis Federation (ITTF);—International Shooting Sport Federation (ISSF);—
World Archery Federation (WA);—International Triathlon Union (ITU);—
International Sailing Federation (ISAF);—International Volleyball Federation
(FIVB); 1.3.2- Other sports governed by other IFs recognised by the IOC]
107. CAS 2015/A/4273
108. Ibid para 40–42
109. Ibid
110. CAS 2015/A/4200
111. Ibid para 7.4
112. Ibid
113. Ibid para 7.8
114. Ibid
115. CAS 2015/A/4163
116. CAS 2015/A/4163 (n 115) para 72
117. Ibid para 94
118. Ibid para 97
119. CAS 2017/A/4984
120. Ibid para 88
121. Ibid para 89
122. Ibid para 123, 125
123. Ibid para 109
124. CAS 2017/A/4984 (n 119) para 123
125. Ibid
126. CAS 2017/A/5016 & CAS 2017/A/5036
127. Ibid para 94
128. CAS 2017/A/5157
129. Ibid para 60
130. Ibid para 57
131. Ibid para 64
132. CAS 2017/A/5296
133. Ibid para 2
134. Ibid para 5
135. Ibid para 37
136. CAS 2017/A/5296 (n 132) para 36
137. Ibid para 55
138. Ibid para 60
139. Ibid
140. Ibid
141. Ibid
142. Ibid
143. Ibid
144. Ibid
145. CAS 2017/A/5296 (n 132) para 60
146. Ibid
147. Ibid
148. Ibid para 83
149. CAS 2017/A/5369
150. Ibid para 147
151. Ibid para 148
152. Ibid para 167
153. Ibid para 164
154. Ibid para 161

155. CAS 2017/A/5392
156. Ibid para 68
157. Ibid para 75
158. CAS 2017/A/5392 (n 155) para 71
159. CAS 2018/A/5581
160. Ibid para 63
161. Ibid para 62
162. Ibid para 68
163. Ibid para 81
164. Ibid
165. CAS 2019/A/6213
166. Ibid para 65
167. Ibid
168. Ibid para 66

References

- James B. Perrine, "Market Solutions to Olympic Problems: Do Athletes, Networks, and Sponsors Really Need the IOC?" *The University of New South Wales Law Journal*, vol. 22, 1999, p. 870
- Olympic Charter, Rule 1-Composition and General Organization of the Olympic Movement (clause 2) [The Three Main Constituents of the Olympic Movement Are the International Olympic Committee ("IOC"), the International Sports Federations ("IFs") and the National Olympic Committees ("NOCs")
- Michael S. Straubel, "Doping Due Process: A Critique of the Doping Control Process in International Sport" *Dickinson Law Review*, vol. 106, 2001–2002, p. 523
- Graham Scambler, "Sociology, Sport and Change: 1-Ancient to Modern" www.grahamscambler.com/sociology-sport-and-change-1-ancient-to-modern/ (accessed 10th January 2021)
- James H. Frey and D. Stanley Eitzen, "Sport and Society" *The Annual Review of Sociology*, vol. 17, 1991, pp. 503–522
- Stefan Szymanski, "A Theory of the Evolution of Modern Sport" *Journal of Sport History*, vol. 35, no. 1, 2008, pp. 1–32. JSTOR www.jstor.org/stable/26404949 (accessed 2nd February 2021)
- Paavo Seppänen, "The Idealistic and Factual Role of Sport in International Understanding" *Current Research on Peace and Violence: Sports Relations & International Understanding*, vol. 5, no. 2–3, 1982, pp. 113–121. JSTOR www.jstor.org/stable/40724935 (accessed 2nd February 2021)
- Helen Jefferson Lenskyj, *Gender Politics and the Olympic Industry* (Palgrave Pivot, 2013)
- Association of IOC Recognised International Sports Federations, "About Arisf—Who We Are" www.arisf.sport/who-we-are.aspx (accessed 13th January 2021)
- International Olympic Committee, "Recognised Organisations" www.olympic.org/ioc-governance-affiliate-organisations (accessed 13th January 2021)
- Kurt Badenhausen, "How a Sport Becomes an Olympic Event" *Forbes* www.forbes.com/sites/kurtbadenhausen/2016/08/09/how-a-sport-becomes-an-olympic-event/?sh=295e5a3c2ce9 (accessed 13th February 2021)
- Global Association of International Sports Federations (GAISF), "Members" https://gaisf.sport/members/ (accessed 14th February 2021)

- "AIMS" http://aimsisf.org/about-aims/ (accessed 14th February 2021)
- "World Anti-Doping Code 2015 with 2019 Amendments" www.wada-ama.org/sites/default/files/resources/files/wada_anti-doping_code_2019_english_final_revised_v1_linked.pdf (accessed 1st February 2021)
- Lovely Dasgupta, *The World Anti-Doping Code-Fit for Purpose?* (Routledge 2019)
- "World Anti-Doping Code 2021" www.wada-ama.org/sites/default/files/resources/files/2021_wada_code.pdf (accessed 1st February 2021)
- Proposed Changes to Provisions in 2015 World Anti-Doping Code Relating to Compliance by Signatories, "2015 World Anti-Doping Code Amendments Adopted by Wada's Foundation Board on 16 November 2017 and to Come into Force on 1 April 2018" www.wada-ama.org/sites/default/files/2015_code_november2017_amendments_en.pdf (accessed 15th February 2021)
- "Amendments to Article 7.4 of the Code Accepted by the World Anti-Doping Agency's Foundation Board on 16 May 2019 and to Come into Force on 1 June 2019" www.wada-ama.org/sites/default/files/resources/files/wada_article_7.4_modifications_en.pdf (accessed 15th February 2021)
- "Significant Changes Between the 2009 Code and the 2015 Code, Version 4.0" www.wada-ama.org/sites/default/files/wadc-2015-draft-version-4.0-significant-changes-to-2009-en.pdf (accessed 15th February 2021)
- "World Anti-Doping Code International Standard Code Compliance by Signatories April 2018" www.wada-ama.org/sites/default/files/resources/files/isccs_april_2018_0.pdf (accessed 15th February 2021)
- Court of Arbitration for Sport, "Database" www.tas-cas.org/en/jurisprudence/archive.html (accessed 16th February 2021)
- www.wada-ama.org/sites/default/files/resources/files/international_standard_isccs_2020.pdf (accessed 15th February 2021)
- World Anti-Doping Agency, "Resources List" www.wada-ama.org/en/resources/search?f%5B0%5D=field_topic%3A138&f%5B1%5D=field_resource_type%3A125 (accessed 15th February 2021)
- CAS 2015/A/3899
- "World Anti-Doping Code 2021" www.wada-ama.org/sites/default/files/resources/files/2021_wada_code.pdf (accessed 16th February 2021)
- CAS 94/129
- CAS 2015/A/4273
- CAS 2015/A/4200
- CAS 2015/A/4163
- CAS 2017/A/4984
- CAS 2017/A/5016 & CAS 2017/A/5036
- CAS 2017/A/5157
- CAS 2017/A/5296
- CAS 2017/A/5369
- CAS 2017/A/5392
- CAS 2018/A/5581
- CAS 2019/A/6213

3 Anti-Doping and American Football—Pro Versus Amateur Dichotomy

Introduction

This chapter inquiries into the prevalence of doping within American football and the role played by the International Federation of American Football (IFAF). American football presents a peculiar instance within the narrative on Non-Olympic sports. The sport is split into amateur and professional. And the trajectory of anti-doping compliances within the two is equally divergent. The sport presents a compelling study into the effectiveness of the World Anti-Doping Agency (WADA) Code and its anti-doping program. Importantly, this chapter builds upon the argument professed in the previous chapter, viz., there is laxity in enforcement of anti-doping program within the Non-Olympic sports. American football is a good example to substantiate the above point. The sport has faced criticism for its lax attitude toward anti-doping enforcements. However, the same does not seem to have any effect. This chapter begins by introducing the two ends of this sport, viz., amateur and professional football. The next section of the chapter analyzes the anti-doping trajectory within these two ends. A comparison is made between the anti-doping measures within the professional sphere and its amateur counterpart. The chapter then goes onto analyzing the anti-doping cases, as reported in the media and debated before the Court of Arbitration for Sports (CAS). The tussle between the USA and other members of IFAF on anti-doping measures is discussed herein. The chapter then goes onto critique the criterion that WADA and International Olympic Committee (IOC) had applied for granting recognition to IFAF and looks into the role of the WADA and the IOC in view of lapses by IFAF in effective enforcement of the Code. This chapter also inspects the interrelationship between NFL and IFAF and the anti-doping narrative they both support and promote. This chapter argues that IFAF and NFL anti-doping controversies challenge the homogenization process of WADA. Finally, this chapter insists that the continued recognition of IFAF and the relatively benign reaction of both IOC and WADA have everything to do with the bargaining power of the members.

DOI: 10.4324/9781003082309-3

American Football—The Professional Versus Amateur Split

American football originated from the modifications introduced by the Americans to the Rugby rules. As per David Riesman and Reuel Denney

> [t]he Americans . . ., set in motion a redesign of the game [Rugby]. . . . Emphasis completely shifted from the kicking game; it also shifted away from the combined kicking and running possible under Rugby rules; it shifted almost entirely in the direction of an emphasis on ball-carrying.[1]

The sports were played exclusively by the college students. As per Tony Collins "Football emerged in the United States in the 1860s and 1870s as a direct consequence of the increasing importance that physical training and sport were acquiring in educational philosophy across anglophone countries."[2] And this link between students and American football was sought to be strengthened by outlawing all forms of professional play. Walter Camp, regarded as "the single individual responsible for the development of American football . . . was a staunch advocate of amateurism . . . ."[3] The Inter-Collegiate Football Association (IFA), founded in the year 1873, passed a resolution in the year 1889 barring the participation of professional players. And the resolution also barred all kinds of payments to amateur players.[4] These changes, however, could not prevent the growth and eventual success of professional American football.

American football's popularity moved beyond colleges and amateurs. It was increasingly being played by the athletic clubs. However, considering the strictures against professional players, the athletic clubs continue to promote amateurism. However, with competition increasing among these clubs, it became difficult to sustain amateurism. The clubs started finding ways to subvert the rules against professional players. Accordingly, the clubs competed among themselves to roll out the incentives. These incentives were designed to attract the best players. The star players were given job offers and there was a distribution of trophies and watches for the players after the games.[5] One of the first recorded instances of a professional player involved in the game is dated November 12, 1892.[6] William "Pudge" Heffelfinger became officially the first player to be paid for playing the game. He was formally paid by the Allegheny Athletic Club, or "The Three A's" a sum of 500$.[7] That set the ball rolling for the other clubs and professional football was born. The professional games were ultimately organized into leagues.[8] The teams that played the professional games eventually came together in 1920 to form the American Professional Football Conference (APFC).[9] And the league which these teams were part of was rechristened as American Professional Football Association (APFA).[10] Eventually, on June 24, 1922, the APFA was renamed as National Football League (NFL).[11]

The NFL is arguably the most popular professional sports league within the USA.[12] However, the growth of professional football in America did not dim the popularity of amateur sports. And it is not surprising that both versions of the game continue to enjoy huge popularity till date.[13] From the perspective of the ensuing discussion on Non-Olympic sports, however, it is the amateur version that is relevant. For internationally too, the amateur version is the one that appears to have attracted maximum participation.[14] Canada became one of the first countries, outside the USA, to establish a federation of American football.[15] Subsequently, the sports found their takers in Asia as Japan lead the way.[16] And since then the sports have grown phenomenally across the Globe.[17] The growing popularity of the sport led to the formation of the International Federation of American Football (IFAF). IFAF was granted provisional recognition by the IOC in 2013.[18] In the next year, viz., 2014, IFAF was included as a member of the ARISF. Currently, IFAF is the only recognized federation for American football. It has around 64 National Federations under its governance.[19] And that makes IFAF a considerably powerful IF within the pantheon of Non-Olympic sports.

The role of IFAF in dealing with anti-doping issues is thus an important case study. More so because IOC has granted provisional recognition to IFAF.[20] As per point number 7 of Rule 3 of the IOC Charter (Charter) the "[p]rovisional recognition, or its withdrawal, is decided by the IOC Executive Board for a specific or an indefinite period."[21] The Charter, however, does not give any details as to the ground for granting provisional recognition to an IF, as opposed to full recognition. This ambiguity continues within the ASSOCIATION OF IOC RECOGNISED INTERNATIONAL SPORTS FEDERATIONS (ARISF) Statutes. Article 7 of the ARISF Statutes prescribes IOC recognition as the only criterion for being eligible for membership of ARISF. No distinction is made between full versus provisional recognition of an IF by the IOC.[22] This creates a scenario where provisional recognition does not mar the reputation of a Non-Olympic sport. Further, the ARISF is committed to support the inclusion of its members in the Olympic Program.[23] Thus, the compliance issues pertaining to the WADA Code remain unaddressed. For neither the IOC nor the ARISF seems interested in ensuring effective compliance by the IFAF. And since the professional version of the sport is completely outside the ambit of both IOC and ARISF, it is a freefall for doping. Interestingly, however, IFAF and NFL have close collaboration in furthering the popularity of the sport. Hence, the doping record of IFAF and NFL does make for an important study.

IFAF, NFL, and Doping—Studying the Trajectory

IFAF, being a member of the ARISF, is a signatory to the WADA Code.[24] Accordingly, IFAF has adopted the WADA Code.[25] All the provisions pertaining to the definition of doping, categories of Anti-Doping rule violations (ADRV), establishing the proof of doping or rebutting the same, prohibited list, Therapeutic Use Exemption (TUE), Testing and Investigations, Athlete Whereabouts *et al* are adopted without any modifications.[26] Similarly, WADA

Code provisions pertaining to sample analysis, result management, and sanctions have also been adopted as it is.[27] Finally, the provisions relating to the appeal and limitations period also is same as those in the WADA Code.[28] The point is that IFAF, on paper, has complied with all the mandatory provisions of the WADA Code. However, when it comes to compliance in practice, the story is bleak.[29] The foremost evidence of the said laxity can be gathered from the lack of any reported cases on doping. As argued in the preceding chapter, lack of cases is evidence of lack of compliance. For the sports that proactively enforce the WADA Code will promptly deal with anti-doping violations. Therefore, it is logical to deduce that absence of a reported case on doping raises doubt about the governance of IFAF. IFAF has had issues with governance leading up to a dispute before the Court of Arbitration for Sports (CAS). In the *International Federation of American Football (IFAF), USA Football, Football Canada, Japanese American Football Association (JAFA), Panamanian Federation of American Football & Richard MacLean v. Tommy Wiking*,[30] the presidency of Mr. Tommy Wiking was challenged.[31]

Mr. Wiking was elected as IFAF President from 2006 to 2016.[32] On February 3, 2015, Mr. Wiking submitted his resignation from the said post, citing health grounds.[33] The said resignation was accepted on February 4, 2015.[34] The said decision of the Executive Board of the IFAF was notified to Mr. Wiking on February 6, 2015.[35] The said resignation was to take effect from April 30, 2015.[36] However, Mr. Wiking disputed his resignation[37] and challenged the decision of the IFAF to elect a new president.[38] There was thus a leadership crisis within IFAF with Mr. Wiking and his supporter legally challenging the IFAF's decision.[39] Eventually, the matter landed up before CAS with both the parties blaming each other for the mess.[40] The IFAF and its supporters pleaded that CAS should

> [d]eclare that Mr. Wiking resigned as President of IFAF on 3 February 2015 and that this was accepted by IFAF; (ii) Declare that the IFAF Congress held in Ohio on 17 July 2015 in which Mr. Roope Noronen was elected as interim President was the only legitimate IFAF Congress held on that date; (iii) Declare that any actions by the rogue-IFAF lead by Mr. Wiking are null and void; (iv) Declare that Mr. Richard MacLean was duly elected as President of the IFAF in the Congress held in New York on 17 September 2016; (v) Order that Mr. Wiking cease and desist from acting as and referring to himself as the President of IFAF; (vi) Order that Mr. Wiking shall bear all the arbitration costs and reimburse the Claimants for any advance on such costs, including the filing fee; Order Mr. Wiking to reimburse the Claimants' legal fees and other expenses related to the present arbitration.[41]

Mr. Wiking in return pleaded that CAS should

> [d]ismiss in their entirety any and all requests for relief submitted in the Request for Arbitration and in the Statement of Claim . . . Order the

Claimants to bear all arbitration costs and to reimburse Mr. Wiking's legal fees and other expenses related to the present arbitration.[42]

CAS, upon a detailed analysis of the entire set of facts and evidence, upheld the contention of IFAF. CAS declared that the

> Panel concludes that Mr Wiking validly resigned as President of IFAF on 3 February 2015. . . . Consequently, Mr Wiking's resignation automatically became effective on 30 April 2015. . . . His late change of mind about this could not affect the clear legal situation and is thus irrelevant. His presidency . . . ended on 30 April.[43]

At present IFAF is headed by Richard MacLean who has ensured that the internal disputes and disruptions are kept at bay.[44] However, only time will tell whether history will repeat itself or not. IFAF's history shows that strife relating to governance is not new and the dispute in 2017 was not the first of its kind. In 2012 too, dispute relating to the governance of the sport by the IFAF had arisen. The dispute arose out of a proposal to undertake "wide-ranging changes to the organisational structure of the IFAF."[45] As part of these extensive changes, the IFAF proposed to

> to eliminate . . . previously independent corporate bodies, the Continental Federations, each of which had been (or would be) organized under the laws of the respective countries in which they were domiciled. Their function as coordinating bodies interposed between the IFAF and the national federations was to be dropped.[46]

This would result in the elimination of the European Federation of American Football (EFAF), a continental governing body of American football in Europe. It would also lead to the elimination of the Asian counterpart of the EFAF. These

> were to be replaced by internal, fully integrated committees responsible directly to the IFAF management. Three new Continental Executive Committees would be created, thus bringing the total to five: IFAF Africa, IFAF Americas, IFAF Asia, IFAF Europe and IFAF Oceania.[47]

At the 15th IFAF Congress on July 5, 2012, the resolution adopting the said proposal was adopted.[48] Consequently, EFAF challenged the said resolution and sought to

> to nullify the adoption of the resolution on the grounds that the Congress . . . violated the substantive membership guarantees accorded to all members of IFAF resulting in the de facto exclusion of the EFAF and . . . ignored the qualified quorum rules.[49]

CAS, after analyzing the arguments and the counter-arguments, declared that the

> termination of EFAF's status as an affiliated member . . . is the result of an organisational change within the IFAF which has affected all of the Continental Federations as affiliated members. . . . The Panel fails to see, however, how EFAF was deprived of its fundamental rights.[50]

This decision highlights the internal dissensions that IFAF had to handle.[51] Though currently there appears to be no governance issue bogging IFAF,[52] this does not seem to have improved its anti-doping measures. IFAF's continuing association with the NFL further explains its lax attitude toward Code compliance. Understandably collaboration with the NFL is beneficial for the promotion of sports. However, this association does not inspire any faith in the intention of IFAF. This suspicion about IFAF's willingness to stringently comply with the Code is justified. For the NFL has an abysmal record in anti-doping measures. Importantly so because NFL's anti-doping measures are not dictated by the WADA Code. As mentioned earlier, NFL is outside the ambit of IOC as well as WADA.[53] Since it represents the professional version of American football, the anti-doping rules are customized as per its requirements. The reason for this blatant divergence from the WADA Code is that NFL is not a signatory to the WADA Code.[54] The NFL anti-doping Code is thus exclusively the outcome of the Collective Bargaining Agreement (CBG) with its players.[55] And that ensures that the anti-doping policy is geared toward accommodating the interests of the players.

Incidentally, NFL has been the first sports professional league in the USA to adopt an anti-doping policy as early as 1987.[56] Its anti-doping policy is the most stringent among all the professional sports leagues in the USA.[57] However, the current anti-doping policy, as incorporated in the CBA is excessively benign as compared to the Code.[58] The policy of the NFL is geared toward providing clinical treatment and care as well as support to players involved in doping.[59] This approach favors rehabilitation as opposed to imposing punitive sanctions on the guilty. There is thus a fundamental divergence in the philosophy of the WADA Code and the NFL policy. This is evident from the fact that the provision dealing with doping is part of the Article on "PLAYERS' RIGHTS TO MEDICAL CARE AND TREATMENT."[60] And Section 9 of the said Article declares that the

> [p]arties agree that substance abuse and the use of performance-enhancing substances are unacceptable within the NFL, and that it is the responsibility of the Parties to deter and detect the use of performance-enhancing substances and to offer programs of intervention, rehabilitation, and support to players who have substance abuse problems.[61]

In contrast, the Code incorporates the strict liability principle.[62] The rigor of the Code is further enhanced through stringent sanctions.[63] This stringency has been detrimental to the Olympic athletes, threatening their careers.[64] However, NFL's liberal policy on doping, on the other hand, treats the guilty as victims and not as a perpetrator.[65] This liberal policy of the NFL when read with the anti-doping commitments undertaken by the IFAF creates a paradox.

The IFAF is committed to stringently comply with the WADA Code as a condition precedent to being recognized by the IOC.[66] Hence, the continued association with NFL is in clear violation of this commitment. For this association of the IFAF with a sports body having a completely divergent stance on doping undermines the legitimacy of WADA. This is more so because NFL is constantly plagued by cases of doping.[67] However, due to its liberal anti-doping policy, there is no deterrence for the players.[68] The blatant use of performance-enhancing substance within the NFL[69] should have put an end to all collaboration with the IFAF. However, this is not the case. Thus, the continued collaboration between IFAF and NFL puts a question mark on the recognition process of IOC. It also leads to a firm belief that getting recognized by the IOC as a Non-Olympic sport has nothing to do with Code compliance. The collaboration between IFAF and NFL also means that there will be space for doping in the amateur version of the sport. For IFAF's approach toward NFL indicates that it is comfortable ignoring the doping record of the NFL. It can be safely argued then that IFAF will be equally comfortable in ignoring its doping violations. For an IF that is serious about its compliance record will shun all company that fails to deter doping. The response of IOC, WADA, and other IFs to the Russian doping scandal is a clear example of the same.[70] And Russia continues to face the heat of the scandal till date.[71] And this problematizes the response of IFAF to the doping scandals that have afflicted it. The response is neither effective nor wide-ranging. Unsurprisingly, its response toward doping scandals afflicting NFL too is mute.

Doping Controversies—IFAF's Response Muted

On December 27, 2015, Liam Collins, a journalist with the Investigative Unit of Al Jazeera, uncovered the extensive use of performance-enhancing drugs in the NFL.[72] The investigation also revealed that doping was equally prevalent in baseball, the other popular professional sports of the USA.[73] Though NFL vehemently denied the allegations and denounced the report, such denials were not convincing.[74] Al Jazeera stuck to its report[75] and asserted it to be the true representation of facts.[76] The report had its desired effect forcing the NFL to issue a public statement regarding the charges made therein.[77] The revelations are important because the doping allegations in NFL are no longer the concern of the USA alone. NFL has been successfully established as a global sport; hence, the doping issues have wider repercussions.[78] An increasing incidence of doping in the professional sport will lead to diminishing its appeal to consumers outside the USA.[79] And that will be detrimental to the business of the NFL.[80] Hence, the Al Jazeera report is definitely relevant to understand the extent of the doping problem within the NFL.[81] The response of IFAF to the doping scandal within the NFL, however, has been disappointing to say the least. And this is more so in view of the fact that IFAF has close ties with the NFL. The IFAF actively supports the International Player Pathway Program (IPPP) of the NFL. IPPP has been designed and developed by NFL to increase its base across the globe. The IPPP is open to non-USA and non-Canadian athletes with no experience of playing the game as an amateur at the college level.[82]

Since 2017 NFL through the IPPP has sourced in foreign players who are part of the IFAF governed system. Thus, IFAF's cooperation and support are key to the success of the IPPP. In 2021, a press release on the website of IFAF proudly announces the success of the IPPP. As per the press note, IFAF announced that "[e]leven athletes from nine countries will compete for a spot in the 2021 International Player Pathway Program, the NFL announced today. . . . The whole IFAF community is cheering them on and sharing their hopes and expectations."[83] On the same note, Damani Leech, NFL Chief Operating Officer of International, announced that "[w]e look forward to providing athletes from around the world with the opportunity to showcase their skills as we continue to grow the game globally."[84] IFAF's president, Richard MacLean, in the same press release announced that

> The international game has a wealth of talent and we look forward to watching the progress of these players in the coming months as they look to carve a career in the NFL. Their stories will hopefully inspire other players around the world.[85]

Against this background, the stance of IFAF vis-à-vis doping allegations within the NFL also defines their own position on the issue. So far nothing of significance has been done by the IFAF to enhance the belief in their commitment toward Code compliance. Their recognition by the IOC has not made them any more reformed than the NFL.

This is evident from the faux pas that IFAF was involved in with the Global Association of International Sports Federations (GAISF). In 2017, GAISF suspended IFAF for nonpayment of dues for anti-doping services rendered by GAISF.[86] The suspension letter was copied to both IOC and WADA. IFAF primarily faced this problem due to its internal strife and the resulting problem in governance. As noted earlier, the same has been resolved through CAS.[87] However, the point is that IFAF's approach toward anti-doping measures is not clear or evident. Though the current governance measures taken by the IFAF appear to have been appreciated by GAISF in its report,[88] there is no clarity on IFAF's stance vis-à-vis Code compliance. GAISF's report also does not specifically note anything on IFAF's record vis-à-vis Code compliance. Further, IFAF's website too does not give any information on the anti-doping record of its members or the players. It only has information on the anti-doping policy and anti-doping Therapeutic Usage Exemptions (TUEs) form.[89] The only other information available on the IFAF website is about WADA Code and its commitment to ensure a doping-free sport.[90] On the other hand, NFL continues to be in the news for the anti-doping violations of its players.[91]

These points lead one to deduce that being a Non-Olympic sport, IFAF continues to be lax in its Code compliance. The lack of data definitely can be regarded as a lack of monitoring on the part of WADA. It also indicates a lack of reporting on the part of IFAF. With governance issues settled for the present, it needs to be seen whether IFAF's compliance efforts vis-à-vis the Code compliance improves in due course. For it cannot be an argument that professionals dope and amateurs don't.[92] Hence, it cannot be concluded that NFL is always on the wrong side of doping, and IFAF is the good boy of American football. The argument is not that IFAF must be hiding its data on doping. First, trying to argue here is that IFAF is following the trend of Non-Olympic sports. And that relates directly to the concerns raised in the previous chapter, viz., Non-Olympic sports have it easy. Their status as Non-Olympic sports allows them to fall under the radar. They face lesser scrutiny than the Olympic sports. There is a lack of stringent scrutiny at the pre-recognition stage. Neither does the IOC have any mechanism to check their compliance level at the postrecognition stage. IFAF's status of provisional recognition can be at best explained as the outcome of its internal strife. The moment the governance issues are resolved and things are carried on smoothly, IFAF should be able to graduate to fully recognized sports. However, this is not going to address the lack of monitoring at the stage of granting recognition. And that is a loophole that allows IFAF like its other Non-Olympic sports counterparts to be lax on Code compliance.

WADA, IOC, and IFAF—The Ambiguity Persists

The lack of scrutiny on the part of WADA and IOC vis-à-vis IFAF is evident from the treatment meted out to NFL. WADA issued a statement as soon as the Al Jazeera documentary on doping in NFL was broadcasted. The content of the statement substantiates the argument of an inherent dichotomy between Amateur and Professional American Football. WADA expressed its concern about the prevalence of doping in professional sports like the NFL. Further, WADA acknowledged that the professional leagues like the NFL are outside the jurisdiction of WADA. This is so because the professional leagues have not signed up for the WADA Code. However, WADA reiterated its goal of encouraging sports organizations to have a doping-free sport. Accordingly, WADA pointed out that it was making efforts to convince the professional leagues to agree to the Code.[93] WADA specifically referred to NFL and noted that "in particular with the NFL, we have been offering guidance to enhance, and increase the transparency of, their testing program."[94] WADA hoped that there will be a proper investigation into the allegations. WADA concluded by stating that "[w]hile the matter is outside of WADA's mandate; as always, the Agency stands ready and willing to work with authorities as appropriate."[95] This lack of mandate, however, does not prevent WADA from expressing its viewpoint vis-à-vis professional sport in the USA. The same concern seems to be missing in so far as the amateur version of the sport is concerned. Not a single statement appears on the WADA website on IFAF or its anti-doping policy. WADA's role is to monitor, and hence, it needs to clarify the consequence of the association of IFAF with the NFL.

The association of IFAF with the NFL can definitely come under the scrutiny of WADA. As per Article 20.3 of the Code, the recognized IFs have certain specific roles and responsibilities.[96] A perusal of these roles makes it abundantly clear that the IF is required to ensure compliance with the Code. As per Article 20.3.3, athletes participating in a competition/activity authorized by the IF shall have to agree to be bound by the Code as a condition precedent.[97] In the context of the IFAF-NFL arrangement, one can apply the above condition. As per the IPPP,[98] the NFL drafts in players from the IFAF pool. These players are all members of the respective National Federations (NFs). The NFs in turn are members of the IFAF. Hence, IFAF has authority not only over the NFs but also over the players. Thus, before authorizing the players to join the NFL, it has to ensure that the players agree to be bound by the Code. One can argue by stating that the players by being members of the IFAF have accepted the Code. However, reading Article 20.3.3, one can argue that the athletes have to be in compliance with the Code while participating in the authorized competition. It is clear that the IPPP is recognized by IFAF, and players are permitted to join the NFL through the IPPP.[99] IPPP, therefore, can also be termed as an activity authorized by the IFAF. Hence, there is a responsibility upon the IFAF to ensure that the concerned activity and the athlete are in Code compliance.

By failing to follow up the issue of the Code compliance requirement with the NFL, IFAF is clearly violating its responsibilities. Importantly, these responsibilities are imposed on IFAF as a signatory to the Code.[100] Further being a recognized IF, it is also assumed to have agreed to be Code compliant.[101] And as Article 20 is part of the WADA Code, it automatically becomes a responsibility of the signatory.[102] IFAF thus causes breaches of the Code at two levels. At the first and primary level, it is violating its responsibilities by letting NFL get away without implementing the Code. Additionally, by letting the players participate in NFL, it is encouraging them to violate the Code. At the secondary level, it is violating the Olympic Charter by breaching the terms of recognition. For Rule 25 makes it abundantly clear that compliance with WADA Code is a condition precedent to getting recognized by IOC.[103] Additionally, by breaching the Olympic Charter, IFAF is causing IOC to breach its responsibilities under the Code.[104] As stated earlier, it is the IOC that has granted recognition to IFAF. And since Code compliance was a condition precedent to grant of such recognition, IOC is clearly in breach each time IFAF fails to ensure Code compliance. This breach is caused each time a player joins the NFL, from the IFAF pool, and violates the Code. The very basis of the collaboration between IFAF and NFL thus gets problematic. One can argue that IFAF has no authority over NFL or that NFL is not a member of the IFAF.

This argument is tenable considering that IFAF on paper has done nothing to defy WADA. However, if we compare the conduct of IFAF with Olympic sports in general, it appears less stringent in terms of compliance. The collaboration between NFL and IFAF, if analyzed in the context of the Olympic sport, would have led to serious problems. The WADA Code aims at harmonization, and the doping control within Olympic sports is geared toward that objective.

To achieve the said objective, "it is critical for purposes of harmonization that all Signatories base their decisions on the same list of anti-doping rule violations, the same burdens of proof and impose the same Consequences for the same anti-doping rule violations."[105] The current practice of IFAF, however, does not promote harmonization. The attitude of the NFL like all the other professional leagues in the USA is to customize the anti-doping narrative.[106] Accordingly the NFL, as evident from the existing scenario, will continue to defy the WADA and disregard the Code.[107] In such a scenario, the practice of IFAF to support and collaborate with the NFL does not augur well for the harmonization principle. The IFAF by supporting and promoting NFL is undermining the anti-doping narrative. One may critique the current Code on several grounds.[108] However, the practice of IFAF indeed creates an inherently inequitable system for Olympic sports. The entire burden of harmonization thus gets placed on the Olympic sports.[109] One can point out that the IOC is equally responsible for this inequitable system. IOC need not continue with the provisional recognition given to IFAF.[110] Irrespective of the incentives that IFAF has to collaborate with the NFL, it ought to insist on WADA Code compliance as a condition precedent.

In short, it has to be the collective responsibility of both WADA and IOC to force IFAF to take a call on the matter. It is not enough for IFAF to have settled the issue of governance within the sport.[111] Neither is it enough for IFAF to declare that they believe in a doping-free sport.[112] The IOC needs to seriously take note of the collaboration that IFAF has with the NFL. It needs to assert its supremacy and ensure observance of the Olympic Charter.[113] The association with a sport body that does not have stringent anti-doping rules goes against the mandate of the Charter. IOC needs to take a proactive stance in ensuring compliance by IFAF. This is a responsibility that the IOC has to discharge to ensure that parity is maintained between the Olympic sports and the Non-Olympic sports. The reaction of the IOC toward the Russian doping scandal proves that when the need arises, it can be proactive. The IOC constituted two Disciplinary Commissions to investigate the issues that the scandal gave rise to.[114] The investigations pertained to the doping allegations raised vis-à-vis the winter Olympic Games at Sochi. In the case of IFAF, the IOC can conduct a pre-emptive inquiry into its collaboration with NFL. The IOC needs to raise a question as to the manner in which IFAF plans to override the NFL doping problem. The IFAF needs to also answer the question as to how the collaboration conforms to its commitment under the IOC Charter. IOC thus needs to play the role of a sports regulator in its true sense.[115]

The WADA too needs to be equally proactive in its role as the enforcer of the anti-doping program.[116] Once again an analogy can be drawn from the reaction of WADA to the Russian doping scandal. The extent to which it went in ensuring strict sanctions for non-compliance with the Code is exemplary.[117] Similar zeal needs to be shown by WADA in ensuring that IFAF's collaboration with the NFL does not undermine the WADA Code. The collaboration should not be used by the IFAF as an excuse to be lax on its anti-doping measures. Unfortunately, there is complete ambiguity as to the data on Code compliance by IFAF. Hence, WADA has to put in that much effort to ensure that IFAF is constantly monitored. Importantly WADA, with the help of IOC, can conduct suo moto inquiry as to the role of IFAF in promoting NFL's games across the world. For the evidence to that effect can be used to implicate IFAF on the grounds of colluding with the NFL by covertly supporting its anti-doping rules. The allegation of collusion is relevant. Promoting NFL games despite its failure to adopt WADA is a breach on the part of IFAF. And WADA can easily recommend action against IFAF in the form of cancellation of its recognition. For that will make IFAF relook into its collaboration with the professional version of the game. One may even see a change in NFL's attitude toward the WADA Code.

Conclusion

American football's evolution from an amateur activity to an excessively commercialized entity is fascinating. The evolution, however, has not been smooth. At the same time, it has been a learning experience for the people in charge of running the sport. The growth trajectory of the amateur and the professional version of the sport has had an effect on the response toward anti-doping measures. The amateur sports dreams of becoming an Olympic sport one day, and thus, they have promptly adopted the WADA Code. However, there is a symbiotic relationship that the amateur has with their professional counterpart. Hence, IFAF has naturally veered toward collaboration with NFL. The professional league, viz., NFL however has an anti-doping policy dictated by the CBG, and it does not match the standards of the Code. Nonetheless, there continues to be a benign response from both the IOC and WADA toward this collaboration. And consequently, IFAF's collaboration with NFL grows from strength to strength. The non-acceptance of the Code by the NFL ought to have made the IFAF to terminate its association. However, IFAF is dictated by commercial incentives to support and promote NFL's games worldwide. Thus, the entire narrative of anti-doping regulation within the IFAF is dictated by the better bargaining power of the NFL. And the benign response of IOC and WADA to IFAF's clear dereliction is governed by the greater bargaining power of the USA. Hence, the treatment of IFAF re-affirms the point that there is a clear disparity within the world of sports between Olympic and Non-Olympic sports. There is no parity or equality when it comes to applying and enforcing the anti-doping regulations among these two categories. Chapters 4 and 5 further establish this point.

Notes

1. David Riesman and Reuel Denney, "Football in America: A Study in Culture Diffusion" *American Quarterly*, vol. 3, no. 4, Winter 1951, pp. 309–325, 316
2. Tony Collins, "Unexceptional Exceptionalism: The Origins of American Football in a Transnational Context" *Journal of Global History*, vol. 8, 2013, pp. 209–230, 212 doi:10.1017/S1740022813000193

3. Collins (n 2) p 224, 227
4. Roger R. Tamte, *Walter Camp and the Creation of American Football* (University of Illinois, 2018)
5. Brandon J. Smith, "Football Origins, Growth and History of the Game" www.thepeoplehistory.com/footballhistory.html (accessed 17th February 2021)
6. Ibid
7. Christopher Mendez, "How the Pigskin Got Professional" http://pabook2.libraries.psu.edu/palitmap/Football.html (accessed 17th February 2021)
8. Smith (n 5)
9. Ibid
10. Ibid
11. PlexusGroupe, "Ninety-Two Years Ago Tuesday, the APFA Became the NFL" https://profootballtalk.nbcsports.com/2014/06/24/ninety-two-years-ago-tuesday-the-apfa-became-the-nfl/ (accessed 17th February 2021)
12. Ryan Alfieri, "How Popular Can the NFL Become? https://bleacherreport.com/articles/1673054-how-popular-can-the-nfl-become (accessed 17th February 2021)
13. Kevin Seifert, "How American Football Is Becoming a Worldwide Sport" www.espn.in/nfl/story/_/id/15273529/how-american-football-becoming-worldwide-sport-europe-china-beyond (accessed 17th February 2021)
14. IFAF, "Governance-About" www.ifaf.org/governance/about- (accessed 17th February 2021)
15. Football Canada, "A Brief History of Football Canada" http://footballcanada.com/about/about-us/ (accessed 17th February 2021)
16. The World Games, "American Football" www.theworldgames.org/sports/American-Football-74 (accessed 17th February 2021)
17. Global Association of International Sports Federation (GAISF), "International Federation of American Football" https://gaisf.sport/members/international-federation-of-american-football/ (accessed 17th February 2021)
18. Duncan Mackay, "American Football Awarded Provisional Recognition by IOC but Long Way to Go Before It Is an Olympic Sport" www.insidethegames.biz/articles/1017396/american-football-awarded-provisional-recognition-by-ioc-but-long-way-to-go-before-it-is-an-olympic-sport (accessed 17th February 2021)
19. AFI, "IFAF, German Federation Intensify Cooperation" www.americanfootballinternational.com/ifaf-german-federation-intensify-cooperation/ (accessed 17th February 2021)
20. Marc Weinreich, "Olympic Football? IOC Gives Provisional Recognition to International Federation of American Football" www.si.com/si-wire/2013/12/10/international-federation-american-football-olympics-nfl (accessed 17th February 2021)
21. International Olympic Committee, "Olympic Charter-in Force as from 17 July 2020," Rule-3- Recognition by the IOC [7. Recognition by the IOC may be provisional or full. Provisional recognition, or its withdrawal, is decided by the IOC Executive Board for a specific or an indefinite period. The IOC Executive Board may determine the conditions according to which provisional recognition may lapse. Full recognition, or its withdrawal, is decided by the Session. All details of recognition procedures are determined by the IOC Executive Board.] https://stillmedab.olympic.org/media/Document%20Library/OlympicOrg/General/EN-Olympic-Charter.pdf#_ga=2.146884275.520978846.1616082425-1246491425.1616082425 (accessed 17th February 2021)
22. Association of IOC Recognised International Sports Federations (ARISF), "Statutes", Article 7—Membership [7.1 ARISF is composed of IFs that are recognised or provisionally recognised by the IOC according to Article 25 of the Olympic Charter as recognised IFs and whose sports are not full member of ASOIF or AIOWF. International Sports Federations that are not recognized by the IOC as recognised IFs cannot be a member of ARISF. 7.2 Each IF that is recognised

or provisionally recognised by the IOC can affiliate as an ARISF member. IFs seeking ARISF membership must submit a written application to the ARISF President. The ARISF President shall confirm the membership request following verification of the recognition status by the IOC. 7.3 A Member will automatically lose its membership status when one or more of its disciplines are included as full member of ASOIF or AIOWF. A Member will also lose its membership should, for any reason whatsoever, the IOC decide to withdraw that member's recognition.]

23. Ibid Article 5—Objects [5.9 To actively support the inclusion of the sports of its members in the Olympic Program]
24. World Anti-Doping Agency, "Code Signatories" www.wada-ama.org/en/code-signatories (accessed 18th February 2021)
25. International Federation of American Football (IFAF), "Anti-Doping Rules in Effect January 1, 2021" https://ifaf.org/downloads/IFAF%20Anti-Doping%20 Rules%202021%20Final%20(1).pdf (accessed 18th February 2021)
26. Ibid
27. Ibid
28. Ibid
29. AFI, "IFAF Suspended by Global Association of International Sports Federations; Expulsion Next?" www.americanfootballinternational.com/ifaf-suspended-by-global-association-of-international-sports-federations-expulsion-next/ (accessed 18th February 2021)
30. CAS 2017/O/5025
31. Ibid para 4
32. Ibid para 8
33. Ibid para 22
34. Ibid para 23
35. Ibid para 24
36. Ibid
37. Ibid para 27
38. Ibid para 49–52
39. Ibid para 56–59
40. Ibid para 86
41. Ibid para 114
42. Ibid para 116
43. Ibid para 169
44. IFAF (n 14)
45. European Federation of American Football (EFAF), American Football Verband Deutschland (AFVD), Schweizerischer American Football Verband (SAFV), Belgian American Football League (BFL) & Irish American Football Association (IAFA) v. International American Football Association (IFAF), CAS 2012/A/2873 para 2.3
46. Ibid para 2.5
47. Ibid para 2.7
48. Ibid para 2.8
49. Ibid
50. Ibid para 6.30
51. Michael Pavitt, "MacLean Seeks to Re-Establish IFAF After Being Confirmed as President by CAS" www.insidethegames.biz/articles/1062344/maclean-seeks-to-re-establish-ifaf-after-being-confirmed-as-president-by-cas (accessed 18th February 2021)
52. Richard MacLean, "Letter to Nations CAS March 1" www.insidethegames.biz/media/file/99737/IFAF%20letter.pdf (accessed 18th February 2021)
53. Christopher N. Burns, *Doping in Sports* (Nova Science Publishers, 2006)
54. World Anti-Doping Agency (n 24)

55. Timothy Liam Epstein, "NFL Compromises on New Doping, Substances Policy" *Chicago Daily Law Bulletin*, vol. 160, no. 197, October 7, 2014, Collective Bargaining Agreement, NFLPA, https://nflpaweb.blob.core.windows.net/website/PDFs/CBA/March-15-2020-NFL-NFLPA-Collective-Bargaining-Agreement-Final-Executed-Copy.pdf (accessed 15th March 2020)

56. Ryan Reszel, "Guilty until Proven Innocent, and Then, Still Guilty: What the World Anti-Doping Agency Can Learn from the National Football League about First-Time Anti-Doping Violations" *Wisconsin International Law Journal*, 29, 2012, pp. 807, 815

57. Ibid

58. NFLPA, "NFL Collective Bargaining Agreement 2020" https://nflpaweb.blob.core.windows.net/media/Default/NFLPA/CBA2020/NFL-NFLPA_CBA_March_5_2020.pdf (accessed 18th February 2021)

59. Sport Resolutions, "NFL Players Agree to New Collective Bargaining Agreement" www.sportresolutions.co.uk/news/view/nfl-players-agree-to-new-collective-bargaining-agreement (accessed 18th February 2021)

60. NFLPA (n 58) Article 39

61. Ibid Section 9 [Substance Abuse and Performance-Enhancing Substances: General Policy- The Parties agree that substance abuse and the use of performance-enhancing substances are unacceptable within the NFL, and that it is the responsibility of the Parties to deter and detect the use of performance-enhancing substances and to offer programs of intervention, rehabilitation, and support to players who have substance abuse problems. Accordingly, in fulfillment of these objectives, the Parties have agreed upon The Policy and Program on Substances of Abuse and the Policy on Performance-Enhancing Substances, which are incorporated into this Agreement."

62. World Anti-Doping Agency, "World Anti-Doping Code 2021-Article 2 Anti-Doping Rule Violations" [2.1.1 It is the Athletes' personal duty to ensure that no Prohibited Substance enters their bodies. Athletes are responsible for any Prohibited Substance or its Metabolites or Markers found to be present in their Samples. Accordingly, it is not necessary that intent, Fault, Negligence or knowing Use on the Athlete's part be demonstrated in order to establish an anti-doping rule violation.]

63. Ibid Article 9 [Automatic Disqualification of Individual Results- An anti-doping rule violation in Individual Sports in connection with an In-Competition test automatically leads to Disqualification of the result obtained in that Competition with all resulting Consequences, including forfeiture of any medals, points and prizes.]; Article 10- Sanctions on Individuals.

64. Reszel (n 56)

65. Sport Resolutions (n 59)

66. International Olympic Committee (n 21), Rule-25 [Recognition of IFs- In order to develop and promote the Olympic Movement, the IOC may recognise as IFs international non-governmental organisations governing one or several sports at the world level, which extends by reference to those organisations recognised by the IFs as governing such sports at the national level. The statutes, practice and activities of the IFs within the Olympic Movement must be in conformity with the Olympic Charter, including the adoption and implementation of the World Anti-Doping Code as well as the Olympic Movement Code on the Prevention of Manipulation of Competitions. Subject to the foregoing, each IF maintains its independence and autonomy in the governance of its sport.]

67. Talia Backhouse, "Doping in American Football; The Issues" https://medium.com/@taliabackhouse/doping-in-american-football-the-issues-e8b3912ee660 (accessed 18th February 2021)

68. Michael Pavitt, "Why Is Doping in the NFL Viewed as Less Important Than in Olympic Sport" www.insidethegames.biz/articles/1075366/michael-pavitt-why-is-doping-in-the-nfl-viewed-as-less-important-than-in-olympic-sport (accessed 18th February 2021)

69. Thomas Torta, "Doping in American Football-Survey of the Prevalence Rates for the Consumption of Dietary Supplements and Doping Substances Among American Football Players by Means of Randomized Response Technique" www.researchgate.net/profile/Thomas-Torta/publication/325713099_DOP-ING_IM_AMERICAN_FOOTBALL_Erhebung_der_Pravalenzen_fur_den_Kon sum_von_Nahrungserganzungsmitteln_und_Dopingsubstanzen_bei_American_ Football_SpielerInnen_mittels_Randomized_Response_Technique_Bachelor/ links/5b1fa905a6fdcc69745c6e6a/DOPING-IM-AMERICAN-FOOTBALL-Erhebung-der-Praevalenzen-fuer-den-Konsum-von-Nahrungsergaenzungsmit teln-und-Dopingsubstanzen-bei-American-Football-SpielerInnen-mittels-Rand omized-Response-Technique-Bache.pdf (accessed 18th February 2021)
70. Lovely Dasgupta, *The World Anti-Doping Code- Fit for Purpose?* (Routledge 2019)
71. Richard W. Pound, "The Russian Doping Scandal: Some Reflections on Responsibility in Sport Governance" *Journal of Olympic Studies*, vol. 1, no. 1, 2020, pp. 3–21
72. Al Jazeera's Investigative Unit, "The Dark Side: The Secret World of Sports Doping" http://america.aljazeera.com/articles/2015/12/27/al-jazeera-investigates-secret-world-of-sports-doping.html (accessed 19th February 2021)
73. Ibid
74. Al Jazeera America, "Football World Responds to Claims Made in Al Jazeera Documentary" http://america.aljazeera.com/watch/shows/morning-news/2015/12/nfl-reacts-to-claims-made-in-al-jazeera-documentary.html (accessed 19th February 2021)
75. Al Jazeera, "The Dark Side: Recording Backs Up Al Jazeera Report" www.alja zeera.com/sports/2015/12/29/the-dark-side-recording-backs-up-al-jazeera-report (accessed 19th February 2021)
76. Mike Freeman, "Players say the NFL has an HGH Problem, Even If Peyton Manning isn't Part of it" https://bleacherreport.com/articles/2602986-players-say-the-nfl-has-an-hgh-problem-even-if-peyton-manning-isnt-part-of-it (accessed 19th February 2021)
77. Al Jazeera, "NFL Vows Comprehensive Probe into Doping Claims" www.alja zeera.com/sports/2016/1/27/nfl-vows-comprehensive-probe-into-doping-claims (accessed 19th February 2021)
78. Kenzie Shofner, "The Globalization of the NFL" www.unitedlanguagegroup.com/ blog/globalization-of-the-nfl (accessed 19th February 2021)
79. Score and Change, "How the NFL Aims for Globalisation of American Football" www.scoreandchange.com/how-nfl-aims-globalisation-american-football/ (accessed 19th February 2021)
80. Daniel Gandert and Fabian Ronisky, "American Professional Sports is a Doper's Paradise: It's Time We Make a Change" *North Dakota Law Review*, vol. 86, no. 4, 2010, pp. 813–844
81. Bilal Chaudry, "Caught in a Rundown: The Need for a Zero-Tolerance Drug Policy to Bring Integrity Back into Professional Sports and Stop the Spread of Performance Enhancing Drugs into Society" *Hofstra Law Review*, vol. 43, no. 2, Winter 2014, pp. 563–600
82. Bill-in-Bangkok, "The International Player Pathway Program Pays Off for the Redskins" www.hogshaven.com/2020/4/29/21240734/the-international-player-pathway-program-pays-off-for-the-redskins (accessed 19th February 2021)
83. IFAF, "News" https://ifaf.org/news/nfl-player-pathway-program-players-announced (accessed 19th February 2021)
84. Ibid
85. Ibid
86. AFI, "IFAF Suspended by Global Association of International Sports Federations; Expulsion Next?" www.americanfootballinternational.com/ifaf-suspended-by-global-association-of-international-sports-federations-expulsion-next/ (accessed 19th February 2021)

87. CAS 2017/O/5025 (n 30)
88. AFI, "International Federation of American Football Receives High Marks from GAISF" www.americanfootballinternational.com/international-federation-of-american-football-receives-high-marks-from-gaisf/ (accessed 19th February 2021)
89. International Federation of American Football (IFAF), "Corporate Documents" www.ifaf.org/governance/corporate-documents (accessed 19th February 2021)
90. International Federation of American Football (IFAF), "Anti Doping" www.ifaf.org/welfare/anti-doping (accessed 19th February 2021)
91. Brent Schrotenboer, "NFL Player Settles Drug Case vs. His Ex-Trainer Just Weeks Before Trial" www.usatoday.com/story/sports/2020/01/21/nfl-player-settles-doping-case-vs-trainer-just-weeks-before-trial/4527628002/(accessed 19th February 2021)
92. Robert G. Lockie, Matthew D. Jeffriess, Farzad Jalilvand and Samuel J. Callaghan, "A Preliminary Analysis of Supplement Habits, Perceptions, and Information Sources for State Representative Youth American Football Players from Australia" *The Journal of Australian Strength and Conditioning*, vol. 23, no. 7, 2015, pp. 16–24 © ASCA www.researchgate.net/profile/Robert-Lockie/publication/287647787_A_PRELIMINARY_ANALYSIS_OF_SUPPLEMENT_HABITS_PERCEP-TIONS_AND_INFORMATION_SOURCES_FOR_STATE_REPRESENTA-TIVE_YOUTH_AMERICAN_FOOTBALL_PLAYERS_FROM_AUSTRALIA/links/5678a84b08ae502c99d578ab/A-PRELIMINARY-ANALYSIS-OF-SUPPLEMENT-HABITS-PERCEPTIONS-AND-INFORMATION-SOURCES-FOR-STATE-REPRESENTATIVE-YOUTH-AMERICAN-FOOTBALL-PLAYERS-FROM-AUSTRALIA.pdf (accessed 19th February 2021)
93. World Anti-Doping Agency, "WADA Statement on Al Jazeera Documentary" www.wada-ama.org/en/media/news/2015-12/wada-statement-on-al-jazeera-documentary (accessed 19th February 2021)
94. Ibid
95. Ibid
96. World Anti-Doping Agency, "World Anti-Doping Code 2021" [Article 20.3-Roles and Responsibilities of International Federations-20.3.1 To adopt and implement anti-doping policies and rules which conform with the Code and International Standards . . . 20.3.3 To require all Athletes preparing for or participating in a Competition or activity authorized or organized by the International Federation or one of its member organizations, and all Athlete Support Personnel associated with such Athletes, to agree to and be bound by antidoping rules in conformity with the Code as a condition of such participation or involvement . . . 20.3.7 To require each of their National Federations to establish rules requiring all Athletes preparing for or participating in a Competition or activity authorized or organized by a National Federation or one of its member organizations, and all Athlete Support Personnel associated with such Athletes, to agree to be bound by anti-doping rules and the Results Management authority of Anti-Doping Organization in conformity with the Code as a condition of such participation. 20.3.8 To require National Federations to report any information suggesting or relating to an anti-doping rule violation to their National Anti-Doping Organization and International Federation and to cooperate with investigations conducted by any Anti-Doping Organization with authority to conduct the investigation. 20.3.9 To take appropriate action to discourage noncompliance with the Code and the International Standards (a) by Signatories, in accordance with Article 24.1 and the International Standard for Code Compliance by Signatories, and (b) by any other sporting body over which they have authority, in accordance with Article 12.]
97. Ibid
98. Bill-in-Bangkok (n 82)
99. IFAF (n 83)

100. World Anti-Doping Agency (n 24)
101. International Olympic Committee (n 66)
102. World Anti-Doping Agency, "World Anti-Doping Code 2021" [Article 20 Additional Roles and Responsibilities of Signatories and WADA-Each Anti-Doping Organization may delegate aspects of Doping Control or anti-doping Education for which it is responsible but remains fully responsible for ensuring that any aspect it delegates is performed in compliance with the Code. To the extent such delegation is made to a Delegated Third Party that is not a Signatory, the agreement with the Delegated Third Party shall require its compliance with the Code and International Standards.]
103. International Olympic Committee (n 66)
104. World Anti-Doping Agency (n 102) [20.1 Roles and Responsibilities of the International Olympic Committee- 20.1.1 To adopt and implement anti-doping policies and rules for the Olympic Games which conform with the Code and the International Standards. 20.1.2 To require, as a condition of recognition by the International Olympic Committee, that International Federations and National Olympic Committees within the Olympic Movement are in compliance with the Code and the International Standards. . .]
105. World Anti-Doping Agency (n 102) [Introduction]
106. NFLPA (n 58)
107. Liam Morgan, "Two-Week Ban Given to NFL Player Highlights Anti-Doping Issues in US, WADA Claim" www.insidethegames.biz/articles/1101240/wada-hit-out-at-two-week-nfl-player-ban#:~:text=The%20World%20Anti%2DDoping%20Agency,exist%20in%20the%20United%20States%22. (accessed 19th February 2021)
108. Lovely Dasgupta (n 70)
109. Dag Vidar Hanstada, Eivind Å. Skilleb and Sigmund Loland, "Harmonization of Anti-Doping Work: Myth or Reality?" *Sport in Society*, vol. 13, no. 3, 2010, pp. 418–430 www.researchgate.net/publication/233167255_Harmonization_of_Anti-doping_Work_Myth_or_Reality (accessed 19th February 2021)
110. Duncan Mackay (n 18)
111. CAS 2017/O/5025 (n 30)
112. IFAF (n 90)
113. Antoine Duval, "The Olympic Charter: A Transnational Constitution Without a State?" *Journal of Law and Society*, vol. 45, no. S1, July 2018 www.researchgate.net/publication/326496940_The_Olympic_Charter_A_Transnational_Constitution_Without_a_State (accessed 19th February 2021)
114. International Olympic Committee, "IOC Disciplinary Commission Schmid Report.pdf" https://stillmed.olympic.org/media/Document%20Library/OlympicOrg/IOC/Who-We-Are/Commissions/Disciplinary-Commission/IOC-DC-Schmid/IOC-Disciplinary-Commission-Schmid-Report.pdf (accessed 19th February 2019)
115. Marc Zemel, "How Powerful Is the IOC?—Let's Talk About the Environment" https://studentorgs.kentlaw.iit.edu/ckjeel/wp-content/uploads/sites/23/2014/09/v1i2-spring2011-3-Zemel.pdf (accessed 19th February 2021)
116. Emmanuel Macedo, "WADA and Imperialism? A Philosophical Look into Anti-Doping and Athletes as coloniser and Colonized" *International Journal of Sport Policy*, vol. 10, no. 3, 2018, pp. 1–13 www.researchgate.net/publication/324595679_WADA_and_imperialism_A_philosophical_look_into_anti-doping_and_athletes_as_coloniser_and_colonised (accessed 20th February 2021)
117. Lovely Dasgupta (n 70)

References

- David Riesman and Reuel Denney, "Football in America: A Study in Culture Diffusion" *American Quarterly*, vol. 3, no. 4, Winter 1951, pp. 309–325, 316
- Tony Collins, "Unexceptional Exceptionalism: The Origins of American Football in a Transnational Context" *Journal of Global History*, vol. 8, 2013, pp. 209–230 doi:10.1017/S1740022813000193
- Roger R. Tamte, *Walter Camp and the Creation of American Football* (University of Illinois, 2018)
- Brandon J. Smith, "Football Origins, Growth and History of the Game" www.thepeo plehistory.com/footballhistory.html (accessed 17th February 2021)
- Christopher Mendez, "How the Pigskin Got Professional" http://pabook2.libraries. psu.edu/palitmap/Football.html (accessed 17th February 2021)
- PlexusGroupe, "Ninety-Two Years Ago Tuesday, the APFA Became the NFL" https:// profootballtalk.nbcsports.com/2014/06/24/ninety-two-years-ago-tuesday-the-apfa-became-the-nfl/ (accessed 17th February 2021)
- Ryan Alfieri, "How Popular Can the NFL Become? https://bleacherreport.com/ articles/1673054-how-popular-can-the-nfl-become (accessed 17th February 2021)
- Kevin Seifert, "How American Football Is Becoming a Worldwide Sport" www. espn.in/nfl/story/_/id/15273529/how-american-football-becoming-worldwide-sport-europe-china-beyond (accessed 17th February 2021)
- IFAF, "Governance-About" www.ifaf.org/governance/about- (accessed 17th February 2021)
- Football Canada, "A Brief History of Football Canada" http://footballcanada.com/ about/about-us/ (accessed 17th February 2021)
- The World Games, "American Football" www.theworldgames.org/sports/American-Football-74 (accessed 17th February 2021)
- Global Association of International Sports Federation (GAISF), "International Federation of American Football" https://gaisf.sport/members/international-federation-of-american-football/ (accessed 17th February 2021)
- Duncan Mackay, "American Football Awarded Provisional Recognition by IOC but Long Way to Go Before It Is an Olympic Sport" www.insidethegames.biz/arti cles/1017396/american-football-awarded-provisional-recognition-by-ioc-but-long-way-to-go-before-it-is-an-olympic-sport (accessed 17th February 2021)
- AFI, "IFAF, German Federation Intensify Cooperation" www.americanfootball international.com/ifaf-german-federation-intensify-cooperation/ (accessed 17th February 2021)
- Marc Weinreich, "Olympic Football? IOC Gives Provisional Recognition to International Federation of American Football" www.si.com/si-wire/2013/12/10/interna tional-federation-american-football-olympics-nfl (accessed 17th February 2021)
- "International Olympic Committee" https://stillmedab.olympic.org/media/Document% 20Library/OlympicOrg/General/EN-Olympic-Charter.pdf#_ga=2.1468 84275.520978846.1616082425-1246491425.1616082425 (accessed 17th February 2021)
- International Federation of American Football (IFAF), "Anti-Doping Rules in Effect January 1, 2021" https://ifaf.org/downloads/IFAF%20Anti-Doping%20Rules%20 2021%20Final%20(1).pdf (accessed 18th February 2021)
- AFI, "IFAF Suspended by Global Association of International Sports Federations; Expulsion Next?" www.americanfootballinternational.com/ifaf-suspended-

by-global-association-of-international-sports-federations-expulsion-next/ (accessed 18th February 2021)
- CAS 2017/O/5025
- European Federation of American Football (EFAF), American Football Verband Deutschland (AFVD), Schweizerischer American Football Verband (SAFV), Belgian American Football League (BFL) & Irish American Football Association (IAFA) v. International American Football Association (IFAF), CAS 2012/A/2873
- Michael Pavitt, "MacLean Seeks to Re-Establish IFAF After Being Confirmed as President by CAS" www.insidethegames.biz/articles/1062344/maclean-seeks-to-re-establish-ifaf-after-being-confirmed-as-president-by-cas (accessed 18th February 2021)
- Richard MacLean, "Letter to Nations CAS March 1" www.insidethegames.biz/media/file/99737/IFAF%20letter.pdf (accessed 18th February 2021)
- Christopher N. Burns, *Doping in Sports* (Nova Science Publishers, 2006)
- Timothy Liam Epstein, "NFL Compromises on New Doping, Substances Policy" *Chicago Daily Law Bulletin*, vol. 160, no. 197, October 7, 2014.
- Ryan Reszel, "Guilty Until Proven Innocent, and Then, Still Guilty: What the World Anti-Doping Agency Can Learn from the National Football League About First-Time Anti-Doping Violations" *Wisconsin International Law Journal*, 29, 2012, pp. 807, 815
- NFLPA, "NFL Collective Bargaining Agreement 2020" https://nflpaweb.blob.core.windows.net/media/Default/NFLPA/CBA2020/NFL-NFLPA_CBA_March_5_2020.pdf (accessed 18th February 2021)
- Sport Resolutions, "NFL Players Agree to New Collective Bargaining Agreement" www.sportresolutions.co.uk/news/view/nfl-players-agree-to-new-collective-bar gaining-agreement (accessed 18th February 2021)
- Talia Backhouse, "Doping in American Football: The Issues" https://medium.com/@taliabackhouse/doping-in-american-football-the-issues-e8b3912ee660 (accessed 18th February 2021)
- Michael Pavitt, "Why Is Doping in the NFL Viewed as Less Important Than in Olympic Sport" www.insidethegames.biz/articles/1075366/michael-pavitt-why-is-doping-in-the-nfl-viewed-as-less-important-than-in-olympic-sport (accessed 18th February 2021)
- Thomas Torta, "Doping in American Football-Survey of the Prevalence Rates for the Consumption of Dietary Supplements and Doping Substances Among American Football Players by Means of Randomized Response Technique" www.research gate.net/profile/Thomas-Torta/publication/325713099_doping_im_american_foot ball_Erhebung_der_Pravalenzen_fur_den_Konsum_von_Nahrungserganzungsmit teln_und_Dopingsubstanzen_bei_American_Football_SpielerInnen_mittels_Ran domized_Response_Technique_Bachelor/links/5b1fa905a6fdcc69745c6e6a/DOPING-IM-AMERICAN-FOOTBALL-Erhebung-der-Praevalenzen-fuer-den-Konsum-von-Nahrungsergaenzungsmitteln-und-Dopingsubstanzen-bei-Ameri can-Football-SpielerInnen-mittels-Randomized-Response-Technique-Bache.pdf (accessed 18th February 2021)
- Lovely Dasgupta, *The World Anti-Doping Code- Fit for Purpose?* (Routledge 2019)
- Richard W. Pound, "The Russian Doping Scandal: Some Reflections on Respon sibility in Sport Governance" *Journal of Olympic Studies*, vol. 1, no. 1, 2020, pp. 3–21

- Al Jazeera's Investigative Unit, "The Dark Side: The Secret World of Sports Doping" http://america.aljazeera.com/articles/2015/12/27/al-jazeera-investigates-secret-world-of-sports-doping.html (accessed 19th February 2021)
- Al Jazeera America, "Football World Responds to Claims Made in Al Jazeera Documentary" http://america.aljazeera.com/watch/shows/morning-news/2015/12/nfl-reacts-to-claims-made-in-al-jazeera-documentary.html (accessed 19th February 2021)
- Al Jazeera, "The Dark Side: Recording Backs Up Al Jazeera Report" www.aljazeera.com/sports/2015/12/29/the-dark-side-recording-backs-up-al-jazeera-report (accessed 19th February 2021)
- Mike Freeman, "Players Say the NFL Has an HGH Problem, Even If Peyton Manning isn't Part of It" https://bleacherreport.com/articles/2602986-players-say-the-nfl-has-an-hgh-problem-even-if-peyton-manning-isnt-part-of-it (accessed 19th February 2021)
- Al Jazeera, "NFL Vows Comprehensive Probe into Doping Claims" www.aljazeera.com/sports/2016/1/27/nfl-vows-comprehensive-probe-into-doping-claims (accessed 19th February 2021)
- Kenzie Shofner, "The Globalization of the NFL" www.unitedlanguagegroup.com/blog/globalization-of-the-nfl (accessed 19th February 2021)
- Score and Change, "How the NFL Aims for Globalisation of American Football" www.scoreandchange.com/how-nfl-aims-globalisation-american-football/ (accessed 19th February 2021)
- Daniel Gandert and Fabian Ronisky, "American Professional Sports Is a Doper's Paradise: It's Time We Make a Change" *North Dakota Law Review*, vol. 86, no. 4, 2010, pp. 813–844
- Bill-in-Bangkok, "The International Player Pathway Program Pays Off for the Redskins" www.hogshaven.com/2020/4/29/21240734/the-international-player-pathway-program-pays-off-for-the-redskins (accessed 19th February 2021)
- IFAF, "News" https://ifaf.org/news/nfl-player-pathway-program-players-announced (accessed 19th February 2021)
- Bilal Chaudry, "Caught in a Rundown: The Need for a Zero-Tolerance Drug Policy to Bring Integrity Back into Professional Sports and Stop the Spread of Performance Enhancing Drugs into Society," *Hofstra Law Review*, vol. 43, no. 2, Winter 2014, pp. 563–600
- AFI, "IFAF Suspended by Global Association of International Sports Federations; Expulsion Next?" www.americanfootballinternational.com/ifaf-suspended-by-global-association-of-international-sports-federations-expulsion-next/ (accessed 19th February 2021)
- AFI, "International Federation of American Football Receives High Marks from GAISF" www.americanfootballinternational.com/international-federation-of-american-football-receives-high-marks-from-gaisf/ (accessed 19th February 2021)
- International Federation of American Football (IFAF), "Corporate Documents" www.ifaf.org/governance/corporate-documents (accessed 19th February 2021)
- International Federation of American Football (IFAF), "Anti Doping" www.ifaf.org/welfare/anti-doping (accessed 19th February 2021)
- Brent Schrotenboer, "NFL Player Settles Drug Case vs. His Ex-Trainer Just Weeks Before Trial" www.usatoday.com/story/sports/2020/01/21/nfl-player-settles-dop

ing-case-vs-trainer-just-weeks-before-trial/4527628002/ (accessed 19th February 2021)

- Robert G. Lockie, Matthew D. Jeffriess, Farzad Jalilvand and Samuel J. Callaghan, "A Preliminary Analysis of Supplement Habits, Perceptions, and Information Sources for State Representative Youth American Football Players from Australia" *The Journal of Australian Strength and Conditioning*, vol. 23, no. 7, 2015, pp. 16–24 © ASCA www.researchgate.net/profile/Robert-Lockie/publication/287647787_a_ preliminary_analysis_of_supplement_habits_perceptions_and_information_ sources_for_state_representative_youth_american_football_players_from_australia/ links/5678a84b08ae502c99d578ab/a-preliminary-analysis-of-supplement-habits-perceptions-and-information-sources-for-state-representative-youth-american-football-players-from-australia.pdf (accessed 19th February 2021)
- World Anti-Doping Agency, "WADA Statement on Al Jazeera Documentary" www. wada-ama.org/en/media/news/2015-12/wada-statement-on-al-jazeera-documentary (accessed 19th February 2021)
- Liam Morgan, "Two-Week Ban Given to NFL Player Highlights Anti-Doping Issues in US, WADA Claim" www.insidethegames.biz/articles/1101240/wada-hit-out-at-two-week-nfl-player-ban#:~:text=The%20World%20Anti%2DDoping%20 Agency,exist%20in%20the%20United%20States%22 (accessed 19th February 2021)
- Dag Vidar Hanstada, Eivind Å. Skilleb and Sigmund Loland, "Harmonization of Anti-Doping Work: Myth or Reality?" *Sport in Society*, vol. 13, no. 3, 2010, pp. 418–430 www.researchgate.net/publication/233167255_Harmonization_of_ Anti-doping_Work_Myth_or_Reality (accessed 19th February 2021)
- Antoine Duval, "The Olympic Charter: A Transnational Constitution Without a State?" *Journal of Law and Society*, vol. 45, no. S1, July 2018 www.researchgate. net/publication/326496940_The_Olympic_Charter_A_Transnational_Constitution_ Without_a_State (accessed 19th February 2021)
- International Olympic Committee, "IOC Disciplinary Commission Schmid Report. pdf" https://stillmed.olympic.org/media/Document%20Library/OlympicOrg/IOC/ Who-We-Are/Commissions/Disciplinary-Commission/IOC-DC-Schmid/IOC-Disci plinary-Commission-Schmid-Report.pdf (accessed 19th February 2019)
- Marc Zemel, "How Powerful Is the IOC?—Let's Talk About the Environment" https://studentorgs.kentlaw.iit.edu/ckjeel/wp-content/uploads/sites/23/2014/09/v1i2-spring2011-3-Zemel.pdf (accessed 19th February 2021)
- Emmanuel Macedo, "WADA and Imperialism? A Philosophical Look into Anti-Doping and Athletes as Coloniser and Colonized" *International Journal of Sport Policy*, vol. 10, no. 3, 2018, pp. 1–13 www.researchgate.net/publication/324595679_ WADA_and_imperialism_A_philosophical_look_into_anti-doping_and_athletes_ as_coloniser_and_colonised (accessed 20th February 2021)

4 ICC Versus BCCI— Challenging the Anti-Doping Narrative

Introduction

This chapter looks into the prevalence of doping within cricket. The International Cricket Council (ICC) is the governing body of cricket. Considering that the sport has a huge fan following in some of the world's most populous regions, its stand on doping merits attention. This chapter thus analyzes the anti-doping program of the ICC. It begins by analyzing the implementation of the World Anti-Doping Agency (WADA) Code by the ICC. This will facilitate understanding the compliance level of the ICC vis-à-vis the WADA Code. The next section deals with the approach of the ICC's members in dealing with doping allegations within the sport. This will help understand the equation of the ICC with its members on the issue of WADA Code compliance. Importantly, it will establish the extent to which ICC is serious in dealing with doping. Further, it will also explain the efforts of the ICC in ensuring effective compliance with the WADA Code. It will also help in understanding the consequence that the individual members are likely to face in defying the diktat of ICC. It will also help understand the reasons that convinced International Olympic Committee (IOC) to grant recognition to ICC. ICC's anti-doping measures will also help understand its philosophy as a Non-Olympic sport. Considering that Non-Olympic sports, in general, have been lax toward WADA Code compliance, this understanding is important. The latter section then analyzes in detail the equation of ICC with the Board of Control for Cricket in India (BCCI). This study is important since currently BCCI dominates the sport. Hence, it is indeed a powerful member of the ICC. Therefore, the approach of BCCI toward implementation of the WADA Code is relevant and necessary. It is relevant because BCCI's attitude toward the ICC's anti-doping program determines the narrative on the issue. It is necessary for understanding the control of ICC over BCCI. These analyses will also help us understand the effectiveness of the overall governance structure of ICC. It is also relevant in determining the steps that the IOC ought to take to force ICC to enforce the WADA Code stringently. This chapter will also look into the response of the World Anti-Doping Agency (WADA) toward BCCI's anti-doping program. This is needed to understand the bargaining powers that are involved herein. Accordingly, one

DOI: 10.4324/9781003082309-4

needs to look into the bargaining power of ICC as a Non-Olympic sport vis-à-vis the IOC. Similarly, the bargaining power of ICC vis-à-vis WADA is looked into. The same is done to understand the key factors that lead to the adoption of the WADA Code by the ICC. Analysis on similar lines is made to understand the bargaining power that exists between the ICC and the BCCI. The attempt is to understand the conflict area that exists between the ICC and BCCI on the issues of WADA Code compliance. This chapter argues that the ICC versus BCCI tussle on anti-doping measure is an instance of power play. This chapter points out that to access large markets of South Asia, both WADA and IOC continue to ignore the lax anti-doping measures of ICC. The ICC needs BCCI for its existence; hence, the power play here too is based on the bargaining power of the members.

ICC and the Code—More a Pretense Than Substance

Cricket got recognized as a Non-Olympic sport by the IOC in 2010.[1] It is accordingly a member of the Association of IOC Recognised International Sports Federations (ARISF).[2] ICC, like all the other Non-Olympic sports, became a signatory to the WADA Code in 2006.[3] On paper, ICC appears to be in compliance with the WADA Code. The public stance of the ICC on the issues is obvious. It declares that the anti-doping policy of the ICC is geared toward ensuring that

> cricket plays its part in the global fight against drugs in sport . . . [and] ICC continues in its efforts to: (a) maintain the integrity of the sport of cricket; (b) protect the health and rights of all participants in the sport of cricket; (c) keep the sport of cricket free from doping.[4]

Accordingly, ICC has adopted the WADA Code 2021. This is expected since ICC, like any other recognized IF, is required to adopt WADA Code.[5] The ICC Anti-Doping Code declares that ICC has jurisdiction over all the players participating in international as well as domestic matches.[6] It is made clear that the burden of compliance with the WADA Code is that of ICC. In order to meet this responsibility, the strict liability principle has been incorporated, in consonance with the WADA Code.[7] Similarly, the burden of proof too remains the same, viz., balance of probability for the players. And for the ICC and its members, the burden of proof is the comfortable satisfaction of the Panel.[8] Continuing with the WADA Code, the ICC anti-doping policy has adopted the WADA prescribed prohibited list. Similarly, other mandatory provisions, viz., Article 7.7 (Retirement from Sport), Article 9 (Automatic Disqualification of Individual Results), Article 10 (Sanctions on Individuals), Article 11 (Consequences to Teams), Article 13 (Appeals) with the exception of 13.2.2, 13.6, and 13.7, Article 15.1 (Automatic Binding Effect of Decisions), Article 17 (Statute of Limitations), Article 26 (Interpretation of the Code), and Appendix 1—Definitions have been incorporated.[9]

The ICC requires all its players to sign a document, agreeing to be bound by the ICC Anti-Doping Code.[10] This also is geared toward ensuring the effective implementation of the WADA Code. Through the consent form, the player voluntarily accepts the obligations under the WADA Code.[11] Further, the consent form ensures that the authority of the ICC over the player is formalized. Similarly for all doping-related issues, the players agree to be amenable to the jurisdiction of the ICC's Anti-Doping Tribunal.[12] The said consent form also makes the player agree to the jurisdiction of the Court of Arbitration for Sport (CAS).[13] In the further discharge of its obligation under the WADA Code, ICC has prepared a template for its members. The National Federations under the jurisdiction of the ICC are required to adopt this template of the Anti-Doping Code.[14] The ICC has also made available on its webpage, the ICC Whereabouts Regulations effective from January 1, 2021.[15] The No-Advance Notice Out-of-Competition test is based on the International Standard for Testing and Investigations.[16] Accordingly, ICC is to establish an "International Registered Testing Pool (referred to hereafter as the 'IRTP') of Players who have to provide the information about their whereabouts. . . ."[17] Further, ICC may "establish additional pools of Players and/or National Cricket Federations who are required to provide certain whereabouts information to the ICC."[18] Accordingly, ICC has established National Cricket Federation Pool (NCFP) and "a National Player Pool (referred to hereafter as the 'NPP') of Players who have to provide, and/or whose National Cricket Federations agree to provide, the whereabouts information."[19]

The fact that the National Cricket Federations (NCF) has the option of refusing whereabouts information under these Regulations is problematic. For the ICC Regulations clearly specify that the NCFP comprise the NCF who have consented to provide whereabouts information. This automatically gives an advantage to the NCF with greater bargaining power. As such an NCF can leverage an exemption from whereabouts filing through bargain. Further within the NCFP, the ICC has included male players of the 12 ICC full members[20] and female players of "the National Cricket Federations ranked in the top ten of the ICC Women's ODI /Rankings selected as of dates specified by the ICC (the "NCFP Review Date")."[21] The federations included in the NCFP are responsible for providing all the details pertaining to "location, full address, dates, times, overnight accommodation, etc."[22] In addition, the federations included in the NCFP are also required to "provide whereabouts information to the ICC in respect of such Specified Domestic Event."[23] The ICC selects one domestic event from the men's and women's tourney and designates it as a Specified Domestic Event. The selection covers all the members of the NCFP.[24] Accordingly, the concerned NCF needs to report all details pertaining to the relevant Specified Domestic Event under its jurisdiction.[25] Thus, the ICC ensures whereabouts filing for both the International and the domestic circuit. Consequences are also provided for whereabouts filing failure by an NCF.[26] And after undertaking an administrative review confirming the whereabouts filing failure, the ICC records the same as a filing failure.[27]

Where the said administrative review is not demanded/waived, the finding of ICC is conclusive of the filing failure.[28] Upon three filing failures by the NCF within a period of 12 months, the ICC imposes a fine of 10,000 US dollars.[29] Such an outcome for filing failure does not appear to be deterring enough for a rich NCF. Hence, the compliance requirement of whereabouts filing by an NCF is evidently not stringent enough. It automatically means that if there is no strong deterrence for an NCF, the player under its authority too are not affected. On paper though ICC has subjected the players to the same norms as is mandated by WADA vis-à-vis whereabouts information.[30] The player included in the NPP is required to provide the whereabouts information as per the ICC Regulation. The player's responsibility for filing whereabouts differs based on the status of the player. Thus in the case where "the [p]layer will be with his/her relevant National Cricket Federation training for or playing in International Matches,"[31] the responsibility for filing whereabouts information lies with the player's NCF and not the concerned player. This has to be done within a span of 4 weeks during which the concerned Player is training/playing. Similarly for the player participating in Specified Domestic Event "the responsibility for providing this whereabouts information lies with the relevant National Cricket Federation in whose territory the Specified Domestic Event is taking place, not the Player him/herself."[32] On the other hand for players who have not

> during a continuous three month period, (i) played . . . an International Match or a Domestic Match; (ii) participated in a tour with a representative team of his/her National Cricket Federation; or (iii) participated in at least two training sessions per week with any Relevant Team over a consecutive three week period[33]

is himself/herself responsible for filing whereabouts information.

Similarly if a player is included in the NPP "part way through a calendar month, he/she shall be required to submit his/her initial NPP Player Filing for the remainder of the initial month in which he/she is placed in the NPP,"[34] then also the player will be himself/herself responsible for filing whereabouts information. And this obligation continues for the subsequent calendar months till the player is removed from the NPP. In all the cases where the player is personally responsible for the filing of whereabouts information, failure to do so would be treated as NPP Filing Failure. And this failure will lead to a potential NPP Missed Test by the player. The player may also miss the test "if he/she was unavailable for Testing at the times and locations specified" in the NPP filing of the player.[35] The NPP Missed Test will be regarded as a negligent act on the part of the player unless the same is rebutted.[36] And the rebuttal can be by showing that the player "establishing that no negligent behaviour on his/

her part caused or contributed to, or that, despite the player taking all reasonable steps available to him/her, there was a good reason which caused or contributed to him/her"[37] missing the test. Three NPP Filing Failure and/or NPP Missed Test within a period of 12 months will lead to a player being moved into the IRTP.[38] A player included in the IRTP is subjected to greater scrutiny and obligations. Thus, a "[p]layer in the IRTP is required to make a quarterly Whereabouts Filing with the ICC, either through ADAMS or in exceptional circumstances manually."[39] The liability is personal vis-à-vis the player and delegation of the task will not be a defense against failure of whereabouts filing.[40] The filing failure or missed test by a player in the IRTP will be treated as Anti-Doping Rule Violation (ADRV) under the ICC Anti-Doping Code.[41]

In addition to the aforementioned regulations, ICC has also adopted the WADA prescribed prohibited list and testing protocols.[42] They have also accepted the International Standards as developed and notified by WADA.[43] To reiterate its declared position on balancing the interests of the player's vis-à-vis enforcing anti-doping measures, the ICC has accepted the ATHLETE'S ANTI-DOPING RIGHTS ACT (the Act).[44] The Act as the title suggests is "[t]o ensure that athlete rights within anti-doping are clearly set out, accessible, and universally applicable"[45] The Act has been approved by the Executive Committee based on the recommendation of the WADA Athlete Committee.[46] The Act is an amalgamation of the rights as recognized by the WADA Code as well as those recommended by the Athlete Committee. The recommendation of the Athlete Committee is to be treated as a template of best practice for the IFs across the board.[47] Thus, Part One of the Act codifies the rights as conferred through the WADA Code. The athletes are thus conferred with the following rights:

- Equality of opportunity
- Equitable and fair testing programs
- Medical treatment and protection of health rights
- Right to justice
- Right to accountability
- Whistleblower rights
- Right to education
- Right to data protection
- Rights to compensation
- Protected persons rights
- Rights during a sample collection session
- Right to B sample analysis.[48]

This list is, however, is not exhaustive of the rights available to an athlete under the existing rules and regulations.[49] Part Two of the Act incorporates these rights that the Athlete Committee "encourage anti-doping organizations to adopt and implement within their own organizational structures to further enhance the fight against doping, the integrity of the system, and athlete rights within that system."[50] These rights are as follows:

- Right to an anti-doping system free from corruption
- Right to participate in governance and decision-making
- Right to legal aid.

These three rights are non-binding rights within the Act which the athletes hope will ultimately be adopted by the IFs. ICC by including the Act within its anti-doping program appears to have recognized these best practices. However, the actual execution and enforcement of the ICC Anti-Doping program needs to be scrutinized to understand its effectiveness. The same can be done through the decisions given and sanctions imposed.

ICC Anti-Doping Decisions: Two-Step Forward and One-Step Backward

One of the earliest decisions that are documented in the ICC's website is that of Upul Tharanga.[51] Warushavithana Upul Tharanga was a left-handed opening batsman and an occasional wicketkeeper, for the Sri Lankan National Cricket Team.[52] He was a key player in the 2011 World Cup campaign for the Sri Lankan Team. He accumulated 395 runs in 9 matches at an average of 56.42 including two centuries.[53] After the conclusion of the Semi-Final Match during the 2011 World Cup, Tharanga gave his sample for testing. The same was done as per the ICC Anti-Doping Code in force at the time of the 2011 World Cup. The sample tested positive for prednisone and prednisolone.[54] These are glucocorticoids and included in the prohibited list under the WADA Code of 2011.[55] It is to be noted that they continue to be prohibited under the WADA Code of 2021 as well.[56] ICC constituted an Independent Anti-Doping Tribunal for the purpose of hearing the matter.[57] Tharanga had clearly committed an ADRV as a result of the sample testing positive for the prohibited substance.[58] The defense that Tharanga gave is interesting and needs to be looked into. He accepted the ADRV and apologized for the same.[59] He said the substance found, being specified substance, was consumed unknowingly and inadvertently.[60] The source of the substance was a medicinal preparation that the player took orally to treat pain in his right shoulder.[61] Thus, the same was not intended to increase the performance of the player concerned. The player accepted that all the results attained by the player in the 2011 World Cup should be canceled. However, he pleaded that the ban imposed should not be long enough to affect his playing career.[62]

This case was to be decided under the WADA Code 2009. As per Article 10.2 of the 2009 Code, the standard period of ineligibility for an ADRV was 2 years, in case of the first violation.[63] Further, Article 10.4 laid down the criteria for reducing/eliminating the period of eligibility.[64] As per the comment to Article 10.4, a specified substance is a prohibited substance that has more chances of leading to inadvertent doping. Accordingly, the athlete has to prove to the comfortable satisfaction of the hearing panel that the ingestion of such a substance was not intended to increase the performance. In the said comment, examples of such situations are given wherein the lack of intention can be argued. The absence of such an intention is proven where there is a declaration in advance of a medical condition requiring the use of such a substance. The athlete can also argue lack of intention where the usage or the nature of the substance would not benefit the athlete. Further, the argument pertaining to lack of intention has to be assessed against the degree of fault of the athlete. The athlete needs to give reasons convincing enough to explain his/her departure from the expected standard and rationale behavior.[65] Thus, the requirement for reduction or elimination of sanction due to the use of specified substance was stringent under the 2009 Code. It required the athlete to prove that there was no negligence on his/her part. That the actions of the athlete were reasonable and expected in the given circumstances.

Tharanga, while pleading reduction of the standard period of sanction, did not explain why he departed from the expected behavior. The ICC Tribunal too did not undertake inquiries into the fault of the athlete. On the contrary, the Tribunal went into the life story of the player, his humble beginnings, and honest behavior in the past. Hearing his narrative, the Tribunal observed that "the player to be an honest and truthful man of integrity. We accept his account of events. He did not try to embellish or alter his story to deflect or minimise any blame for what happened."[66] The Tribunal then goes on to record the developments surrounding the involvement of an ayurvedic doctor Mr. Eliyantha White.[67] Mr. White was described by the Tribunal, as the most important healer for the Sri Lankan National Team.[68] Mr. White's importance diminished the role of the official physio Mr. Tommy Simsek.[69] Accordingly, the player, like his other teammates, consulted Mr. White for the treatment of his shoulder pain. In fact, during 2011, the player was under the treatment of Mr. White.[70] The player had an unshakeable belief in Mr. White and was in awe of the popularity of Mr. White. He blindly took all the medicines that were offered to him as part of his treatment by Mr. White.[71] The Tribunal did note this lack of precaution on the part of the player.[72] However, the Tribunal decided that the conduct of the player could be justified since he had indeed a known history of shoulder pain. Further that he was known to be taking medicines as prescribed by Mr. White.[73] This aspect satisfies the example given in the comment to Article 10.4, viz., "the Athlete's open Use or disclosure of his or her Use of the Specified Substance; and a contemporaneous medical records file substantiating the non-sport-related prescription for the Specified Substance."[74] The said conclusion would then be a ground to reduce, if not eliminate the sanction period. The Tribunal further accepted the argument of the player "that an athlete cannot intend to enhance sport performance through the ingestion of a prohibited substance unless the athlete is aware that he has ingested the substance in question."[75]

Accordingly, the Tribunal went on to hold that "the player did not intend to enhance his performance by ingesting the liquids provided by Mr White."[76] The Tribunal thus awarded a sanction period of 3 months. At the same time, the Tribunal regretted the imposing of the said period of ineligibility by noting that

> [w]e take into account that the player will not lose any prize money as a result of the agreed disqualification of his results and performance statistics; but he will suffer the less tangible loss of recognition, at least by official cricket sources, of his achievements during the whole of the 2011 World Cup, including centuries against Zimbabwe and England.[77]

And the concern for the plight of the player led the Tribunal to apply its discretion and "backdate the start of the period of ineligibility to 9 May 2011, the day after the player ceased competing."[78] This decision of the ICC Tribunal is problematic and reveals the attitude of the Non-Olympic sports toward the WADA Code. The Tribunal reasoning is completely in contradiction with the fundamental philosophy of the WADA Code. As per Article 2.1.1 of the WADA Code 2009 "It is each Athlete's personal duty to ensure that no Prohibited Substance enters his or her body. Athletes are responsible for any Prohibited Substance or its Metabolites or Markers found to be present in their Samples."[79] Hence to uphold the contention of the athlete that the lack of knowledge about ingesting a prohibited substance is a valid defense is fundamentally wrong. Further, the Tribunal's reasoning pertaining to the player's medical condition is also in contradiction with the purpose of Article 10.4 of the WADA Code. The player did not have any TUE at the time of the 2011 World Cup. Hence to hold that the player's medical condition was in the common knowledge of his teammates and his NCF lowers the burden of proof of the athlete.

Further, the Tribunal's reduction of the sanction period to 3 months defies any logic or reason. Considering that the Tribunal has only considered the rigor of the anti-doping program is not justification enough. Interestingly, the Tribunal in its conclusion permitted either of the parties to appeal to CAS against its decision. However, ICC never appealed and the player understandably did not appeal. In contrast to the attitude of the ICC toward the leniency shown to the player, the Olympic sports IF are more proactive. For example in *Fédération Internationale de Natation (FINA) v. Fabiola Molina & Confederação Brasileira de Desportos Aquaticos (CBDA)*,[80] FINA challenged the decision of the Doping Control Panel.[81] The panel was formed by the Brazilian National Federation (CBDA) of swimming for hearing the matter of an ADRV.[82] The athlete Ms. Fabiola Molina, a Brazilian swimmer of the international level, was found to have consumed a prohibited substance.[83] The substance methylhexaneamine (MHA) is a prohibited specified substance under the 2011 Prohibited List.[84] Hence, Article 10.4 of the 2009 Code was to apply to the case in connection with the reduction/elimination of sanction.[85] Since CBDA was affiliated with FINA,[86] it was bound by the FINA Anti-Doping rules.[87] And the said rules had incorporated the WADA Code 2009. Consequently, the CBDA constituted

Panel applied Article 10.4 as incorporated in the FINA Anti-Doping Rules and reduced the sanction of Molina to 2 months.[88]

FINA challenged the Panel's decision before CAS on the ground that the reduced sanction was unacceptable and unreasonable.[89] It argued that Article 10.4 "is applicable to unintentional doping and therefore has to relate to the measure of negligence of the Athlete which led to the presence of Prohibited Substance, and . . . that Molina fell short of the required standard of behaviour."[90] CAS, in turn, analyzed the facts and the arguments of all the parties and declared that

> under the WADA World Anti-Doping Code (hereinafter referred to as the "WADC") (on which the FINA DC rules are modelled), that the circumstances to be considered in the assessment of the athlete's fault "must be specific and relevant to explain the athlete's . . . departure from the expected standard of behavior.[91]

Accordingly, the Panel held that

> Molina's negligence was not inconsequential: far from doing everything in her power, she blindly relied on her past experience with the online retailer that provided her with the Supplement, did not check on the Internet or seek any kind of advice.[92]

Accordingly CAS held that

> the sanction of two months imposed by the Decision is too lenient. On the basis of Molina's degree of fault and weighing all the relevant specific factors, the Panel concludes that an appropriate sanction would be a period of ineligibility of six months."[93]

This decision exemplifies the settled jurisprudence pertaining to specified substance and sanction. It is clear that the ICC Anti-Doping Panel neither bothered to rebut nor cared to implement the Code requirement while reducing the sanction in the Tharanga case. As per the records available on the ICC website, the leniency shown in the Tharanga case appears to be the norm.

Tremayne Smartt, the West Indian women cricketer, was sanctioned for a period of 5 months for the use of a specified substance.[94] The specified substance found in her sample was furosemide.[95] It is categorized as diuretics and masking agents in the WADA Prohibited List.[96] The ICC constituted Tribunal declared that though the "substance wasn't used to enhance performance or mask the use of another performance-enhancing drug, but that[the player] had failed to satisfy the high levels of personal responsibility implicit upon her as an international cricketer subject to anti-doping rules."[97] This is in contrast with the discussion on the burden of a proof found in the Tharanga case. Nonetheless, one can also argue that the sanction was lenient in view of the admission of the player. Soon after the decision imposing the sanction, Smartt "conceded she did not effectively check the Prohibited List and would have to accept the consequences."[98] Hence the approach of ICC, notwithstanding the Tribunals observation on the burden of proof, is lax. It is also inconsistent and does not lay down any clear picture as to the level of compliance with the WADA Code. For instance, in the case of Yasir Shah,[99] the ICC Anti-Doping Tribunal imposed a sanction of 3 months. It needs to be noted that the substance in this instance was chlortalidone, a specified substance. And as in the case of Smartt, here too the substance was diuretics and masking agents.[100] The other important point is that the decision was rendered under the 2015 WADA Code, which was more stringent than the 2009 Code.[101] In this case, the reasoning again is based on sympathy toward the player.

The ICC Panel held that the player did not take all possible measures available to him for avoiding the consumption of chlortalidone. However his departure "from that standard in the specific and rather extreme and unique circumstances of this case (urgent and stressful circumstances that he considered in good faith to amount to an emergency) was understandable and in part excusable."[102] Accordingly, the ICC Panel declared that this conduct of the player amounted to "No Significant Fault or Negligence" per Article 10.5.1 of the ICC Code, as incorporated from the 2015 WADA Code.[103] Substantiating this conclusion, the ICC Panel further notes that the player has "promptly admitted the anti-doping rule violation once he had established the facts regarding his mistaken ingestion of Chlortalidone,[and] has expressed significant remorse."[104] On the basis of such considerations, the ICC Panel justified imposing a sanction period of 3 months.[105] This leniency is equally applied to ADRV resulting from Non-Specified substances prohibited at all times. In the case of Mohammad Shahzad, the ADRV was due to the presence of Clenbuterol which is "an anabolic agent that is prohibited at all times (i.e., both in- and out-of-competition). There is no threshold under which this substance is not prohibited."[106] However, the ICC Panel hearing the matter continued with its practice of being lenient. Analyzing the conduct of the player for determining the applicability of No Significant Fault or Negligence, it took a pro-player stand. The following points were regarded as being in favor of the player, viz., (a) the player's lack of anti-doping education and awareness about the do's and don'ts; (b) being based in Afghanistan, the player has limited Internet access; (c) player's knowledge of English language is very basic further limited his access to information on anti-doping literature; and (d) player's conduct in seeking the advice of the team physio established his honesty.[107]

On the basis of the aforementioned reasons, the ICC Panel declared that the player has successfully established No Significant Fault or Negligence,[108] under Article 10.5.2 of the ICC Code (as incorporated from the WADA Code 2015).[109] Accordingly, the sanction was reduced from 2 years to 12 months, as per Article 10.2.2 read with Article 10.5.2 of the WADA Code 2015. Since the ICC Anti-Doping Code had incorporated the mandatory provision of the

WADA Code 2015, the ICC Panel's decision was valid.[110] Though the basis of applying such discretion is not convincing. Further such a lenient and lax approach toward ADRV is not available to Olympic sports. And that highlights the existing gap between Non-Olympic sports and Olympic sports. The laxity toward ADRV violations is inbuilt within the systems of the Non-Olympic sports. The primary reason is that these sports are not part of the Olympic Games. Accordingly, there are no compelling reasons for them to be vigilant with the compliance requirement. The non-inclusion within the Olympic Games though does not justify such laxity for it defeats the very purpose of recognition by the IOC. As will be seen next, the ICC has not taken any measures to ensure that its members observe strict compliance. Understandably so since, as the discussion hereinabove show, ICC itself has been excessively lax toward ADRV by its players. And the decision also shows the attitude of the member NCF toward the ADRV of their players. In short, the entire system as curated and regulated by ICC is not conducive to strict compliance with WADA Code.

The ICC System and Anti-Doping—The Members' Viewpoint

As evident from ICC's website, the anti-doping measures of its members have been equally lax barring few instances here and there. Considering that full members of the ICC are all test playing countries, their performance vis-à-vis anti-doping measures is interesting to note. For the full members form the core of the ICC and have an established culture of cricket. They determine and design the governance of cricket. In contrast, Associate members are those who got inducted over the years as they developed an interest in cricket and started establishing a cricketing culture in their respective countries.[111] Among the test-playing countries, the ICC website archives cases from England, West Indies, South Africa, Pakistan, New Zealand, and Bangladesh. India tops the chart in the number of anti-doping cases, as per the ICC website. However, we will deal with BCCI and its response to ADRV in the next section. Herein, we will review the decisions given by the other test playing countries in cases of ADRV. In MR KAZI ANIK ISLAM, the ADRV was found to have been caused due to the presence of methamphetamine (D-).[112] It is a Non-Specified Stimulant under S 6A of the WADA Code Prohibited List.[113] The relevant rules applied by the Bangladesh Cricket Board (BCB) were those incorporated from WADA Code 2015. Accordingly, Articles 2.1[114] and 2.1.2[115] were relied upon to establish the ADRV.[116] However, BCB liberally interpreted the rules on imposition of sanctions, as incorporated from the WADA Code 2015. Accordingly, Article 10.6.3,[117] as incorporated from the WADA Code 2015 was read liberally enough to benefit the player.[118]

The BCB accordingly brought in considerations that enabled it to liberally assess the degree of fault of the player for reducing the sanction. For else, the original period of ineligibility would have been 4 years.[119] A beneficial interpretation as to the degree of fault will reduce the stringency for the player as well as the period of sanction. BCB thus declared that in

> considering [player's] level of Fault, the BCB has considered his youth and relative inexperience, the fact that he did not ingest the Prohibited Substance in an effort to enhance his sport performance, his limited anti-doping education and his prompt admission of the anti-doping rule violation when first notified to him. . . ."[120]

Thus, BCB imposed a sanction of 2 years and conferred a further benefit on the player by backdating the start of the period of ineligibility.[121] Consequently, the decision rendered on July 2020 imposed a sanction of 2 years which was to end on February 7, 2021. Thus effectively, the sanction imposed was for a period of 8 months.[122] In the case of Harrisyn Jones,[123] the Sports Tribunal of New Zealand took an equally liberal stand vis-à-vis the ADRV caused due to the presence of Clenbuterol.[124] The Tribunal while imposing a sanction of 2 years backdated it by 12 months.[125]

The story of the other test-playing countries does not appear to be any different. The decisions given by the domestic tribunals of these NCFs further the liberal narrative vis-à-vis the sanctions. In the case of Kashif Saddique,[126] the sample tested for the presence of prohibited substances, viz., metabolites of nandrolone and stanozolol. These are Non-Specified substances and are absolutely prohibited without any exception.[127] Consequently, the Pakistan Cricket Board (PCB) constituted an Anti-Doping Tribunal to render a decision in the matter. The player pleaded his innocence and lack of intention to enhance performance. Accordingly, the player relied on the defense of No Fault or Negligence.[128] The main contention was that the medicines the player had taken to treat his shoulder injury. The player had no means of knowing, using the utmost diligence, that the medicines will be the source of a prohibited substance.[129] However, the Tribunal was not convinced and declared that the player failed to establish No Fault or Negligence.[130] Accordingly, the Tribunal imposed a sanction of 2 years considering that it was the first offense.[131] The decision of the Tribunal was based on the PCB anti-doping rules, which in turn were, based on the WADA Code 2009. Accordingly, the sanction was imposed as prescribed under Article 10.2 of the WADA Code 2009[132] and incorporated in the PCB regulations. And for a change, the Tribunal, in this case, did not show leniency by excessively backdating the date of commencement of the sanctions. The only thing that was taken note of was the period of provisional suspension while fixing the date of commencement of the ineligibility.[133] However, PCB's approach in the case of Raza Hasan[134] cannot be said to be in compliance with the WADA Code.

Raza Hasan was found to have committed an ADRV in the year 2015, and his sample was tested for Benzoylecgonine (the main metabolite of cocaine).[135]

This is was a Non-Specified stimulant and is banned in-competition.[136] The player was notified of the same and charged with ADRV.[137] He, however, did not respond to the notice, and neither did he make any attempt to defend himself or counter the charges. In other words, the player was completely non-responsive to the findings of ADRV by the PCB.[138] Consequently, the PCB imposed 2 years of sanction on the player, without conducting any proceedings.[139] The sanction, however, was in accordance with the WADA Code 2009.[140] This itself is problematic for the violation was committed in the year 2015 and accordingly ought to have been dealt with under the WADA 2015 Code.[141] And that would have, in the given circumstances of the case, led to the imposition of 4 years ineligibility. Unfortunately, however, the PCB had not updated its rules and was following the old Code. This is clear evidence of laxity on the part of PCB as well as ICC. For the ICC too, here failed to ensure, that its members update their anti-doping regulations as per the latest version of the WADA Code. Hence, as mentioned earlier, the larger picture is that of lax compliance with the WADA Code. The England and Wales Cricket Board (ECB) imposed a sanction of 12 weeks on Abdur Rehman for testing positive for cannabinoids.[142] As per the WADA Prohibited List of 2012, cannabinoids are banned in-competition.[143] And since the case ought to have been governed by the WADA Code 2009, the sanction period ought to have been 2 years.[144]

This is so because the player admitted to have taken the substance, and thus, the degree of fault of the athlete was indeed on the higher side.[145] There were thus no grounds to reduce the 2 years as per Article 10.4.[146] Unfortunately, though ECB was happy to ignore this fact and applied its discretion arbitrarily. In the case of Rory Kleinveldt,[147] a charge of ADRV was framed by Cricket South Africa (CSA) against the player. The player's sample tested positive for cannabinoids, which is a specified substance and banned in competitions, as already mentioned.[148] Thus, the South African Institute for Drug-Free Sport (SAIDS) had to satisfy itself that grounds exist for reduction/elimination of the sanction. As mentioned earlier, as per the WADA Code 2009, the sanction period is 2 years for the first offense subject to mitigating factors.[149] Article 10.4 of the WADA Code 2009 prescribes the mitigating factor for ADRV arising out of consumption of the specified substance.[150] And SAIDS analyzed the evidence as submitted by the athlete to prove the mitigating factors. SAIDS declared that it is "prepared to accept the evidence of the Athlete that he did not smoke the Cannabis with an intention to enhance his sports performance."[151] On the issue of corroboration of the athlete's contention SAIDS held that since

> the Prosecution has not disputed the evidence as presented by the Athlete, his remorse and apology, and applying common sense to the situation, we believe that it is evident that the Athlete did not intend to enhance performance, despite the lack of independent corroborative evidence on this point."[152]

SAIDS then analyzed the degree of fault of the athlete as required under Article 10.4 of WADA Code 2009. This was needed to determine the extent to which the sanction can be reduced. On the said issue, SAIDS declared that

> as a professional athlete he should have been more prudent in this regard—his evidence as to being slightly under the influence is no defence in this regard. The Athlete could have, and should have, refused the drug and as such taken action to avoid the positive test.[153]

The SAIDS thus went on to hold that the athlete

> did not act within the expected standard of behaviour of a professional athlete . . . the Athlete, as a role model has a responsibility to act in a manner that sets an example to minor children . . . There is material fault on the part of the Athlete.[154]

However, despite all these statements, the SAIDS ended up awarding only 3 months' ineligibility period.[155] This again reflects the scenario within the sports of cricket with respect to compliance with the WADA Code. Neither ICC nor the member NCFs appear to be keen on deterring the players against the usage of the prohibited substance/methods. In the case of Odean Brown,[156] the ADRV was caused due to whereabouts failure on the part of the player. The Jamaica Anti-Doping Disciplinary Panel analyzed the arguments of the player explaining the reasons for missing the whereabouts filing. The Panel was not convinced with the reasons given by the player and rejected the same.[157] The Panel held that the player was "familiar with filing whereabouts information as he had so filed before."[158] However, the Panel was in favor of imposing a 1-year ineligibility period as per Article 10.3.2 of the Jamaica Anti-Doping Commission (JADCO). The same was based on Article 10.3.2 of the WADA Code 2015.[159] Article 10.3.2 does provide for the flexibility in imposition of ineligibility. However, that is not available if "a pattern of last-minute whereabouts changes or other conduct raises a serious suspicion that the Athlete was trying to avoid being available for Testing."[160]

The Panel, however, found that the conduct of the player makes him amenable to an ineligibility period in excess of 1 year but lesser than 2 years.[161] This was so because the player could not give any convincing explanation for missing the whereabouts filing. However, there was no evidence of manipulation. Nonetheless, the fact that the player was a full-time cricketer, it was expected that he knew his obligation vis-à-vis filling of whereabouts. Hence, the Panel, in this case, imposed a stringent punishment as compared to other cases analyzed herein. The Panel herein, however, clearly explains the basis of the reduction. It also refers to the settled jurisprudence on Article 10.3.2 to arrive at the conclusions and impose a sanction period of 15 months.[162] On the whole, as mentioned, barring few instances, the approach of the NCFs has been to support the player. The anti-doping infringements, thus, do not always enforce or strengthen the WADA Code or its fundamental principles. Though the cases discussed are of those involving the test playing full members of ICC, they are relevant. For it is the full member whose attitude toward compliance with the WADA Code lays down the roadmap for ICC. The associate members are not in a position to steer the ICC governance or its decision-making process. ICC's survival and authority depend on the actions of the full member. The cricket world is primarily dominated by full members. However, among these full members, there are some who are more equal than the others. The dominant member/s, thus, are strong enough to challenge the authority of the ICC. It is thus important that compliance with the WADA Code is studied from the perspective of the BCCI.

BCCI and Anti-Doping Compliance—Bossing the ICC?

THE BOARD OF CONTROL FOR CRICKET IN INDIA (BCCI) has been a full member of ICC since 1929.[163] Over the years, it has gradually grown from strength to strength to become arguably the most powerful NCF within the ICC.[164] BCCI virtually dictates the going on within the cricket world. Its' power has grown to the extent that it has now become the *de facto* rule-maker rather than the follower.[165] The power comes from the financial clout that BCCI has within the world of cricket. For BCCI contributes approximately 70% of the revenue that the ICC receives from its members. And that spells out power, for the day BCCI stops this contribution, ICC will struggle to exist. The financial clout of the BCCI is great enough to dictate the terms to ICC as to the model of revenue sharing to be followed.[166] The clout of BCCI comes from the immense popularity of cricket within India and the subcontinent. For Indians, cricket is religion and the players are the Gods whom the spectators and viewers are fanatic about.[167] This level of popularity of the sport helps BCCI for India is the second-most populous country in the world.[168] The popularity of cricket in India was powered by television as well as the team's winning performances. The starting point of the growth trajectory is the 1983 World Cup which India won. And that set the ball rolling for the games' administrators in India to make BCCI a cash-rich NCF.[169] The smart investment in broadcasting rights eventually resulted in the most successful and rich domestic league of the game, viz., Indian Premier League. For the 2018–2021 season, BCCI has sold IPL's broadcasting rights for a humongous sum of Rs. 16,347.50 crore.[170] And that explains and underlines the clout of BCCI within ICC.[171]

Over the years, BCCI has repeatedly shown to ICC who the actual boss is and forced ICC to change several of its decisions. For instance, in 2001, BCCI forced ICC to remove former English cricketer Mike Denness from his role as the match referee.[172] He was assigned the role of match referee during the India–South Africa bilateral series.[173] The unpardonable crime committed by Denness was to charge and punish Sachin Tendulkar for ball-tampering. In addition, he suspended five other players, including the then captain Sourav Ganguly for excessive appealing.[174] ICC backed Denness to the hilt but

Jagmohan Dalmiya-led BCCI was adamant. India threatened to cancel the rest of the series.[175] They refused to play the third test until Denness was dropped as the ICC match referee for the series. BCCI even threatened to cancel the upcoming tour of England to India.[176] Eventually, BCCI got the South African Cricket Board (CSA) to support its stand and go ahead with the third test. BCCI and CSA came together and sacked Denness, which further infuriated ICC. ICC withdrew recognition to the third test match as an official match.[177] Nonetheless, BCCI had its way, and ICC could not do anything. ICC backed out from further confrontation with the BCCI on the issue. As for Denness, the controversy ended his career as a match referee. ICC appointed him as a match referee in only two more test matches and three One Day Internationals. And thereafter he was never re-appointed by the ICC as a match referee.[178] The next incident wherein BCCI flexed its muscle vis-à-vis ICC was with respect to the ambush marketing rules.

The ICC introduced an ambush marketing clause that prohibited the players from appearing in the advertisement or endorsing products of rival companies/ brands. In short, ICC wanted to protect its sponsors by ensuring that the players and teams stick with only the official sponsors during multilateral tournaments. Thus, for ICC-sponsored and organized tournaments like the World Cup, players had to follow this norm. Obviously considering the financial gains cricket in India brings in, the Indian players were affected the most. Consequently, the players through BCCI expressed their unhappiness and refused to accept such restrictions. The Indian players through BCCI threatened to boycott the 2003 cricket World Cup unless ICC made an exception for them. ICC ultimately had to bow down to the pressure of BCCI and made an exception in the case of Indian players. Consequently, the Indian players were bound by the ambush marketing clause only for the duration of the tournament. Post the World Cup as well as prior to the commencement of the World Cup, the Indian players were free to endorse rival companies.[179] These are just two of the several instances where BCCI has flexed its muscle to cow down ICC. In a candid conversation with James Astill for his book, Niranjan Shah, former BCCI Secretary, unabashedly glorifies the power of BCCI.[180] As per Shah

> ICC is trying to control us. . . . Most of the other boards do not like that we make so much money . . . their revenue depends on whether our team goes to play them . . . For cricket the only market in the world is India. The market is here. So we will control cricket, naturally.[181]

This statement of Shah sums up the attitude of BCCI towards ICC as well as cricket.

Against this background, one can clearly see that it will be a tad difficult if not impossible for ICC to make BCCI WADA Code compliant. It was indeed the case till August 2019 for BCCI refused to be amenable to the WADA Code.[182] As a consequence, BCCI was using its own discretion in dealing with doping issues involving its player. BCCI, in continuation of its stand against the WADA Code, refused to submit to the jurisdiction of the National Anti-Doping Agency (NADA).[183] NADA is an agency established by the Government of India for implementing the WADA Code within the country. It is also responsible for conduction anti-doping research and education programs and spreading awareness about the WADA Code.[184] BCCI has, however, prior to 2019, refused to be subject to the jurisdiction of NADA.[185] BCCI's resistance came due to several reasons, the primary of which has been whereabouts filing. The elite player of BCCI has had vehemently objected to being subject to the requirement of whereabouts filing. Hence, BCCI was not agreeing to abide by the WADA Code.[186] Additionally, BCCI also argued that since did not receive any funding from the Government of India, it was autonomous. Accordingly, it was outside the jurisdiction of the Government as well as NADA.[187] BCCI also questioned the quality of tests being conducted by NADA and questioned the competency of NADA's personnel. BCCI also questioned NADA's level of efficacy in submitting the test report. BCCI alleged inordinate delay on part of the NADA in completing the sample testing process.[188] BCCI in effect argued that it was outside the systems created by ICC as well as the Government of India. BCCI's argument was primarily based on the fact that it is a private entity and thus is not amenable to the diktats of the Government of India. Importantly, BCCI continues to take a stand that it is not a recognized National Sports Federation.[189] Thus, BCCI's acceptance of NADA in the year 2019 needs to be viewed skeptically. For the same might lead to any fundamental change in the attitude of BCCI toward WADA Code compliance.

BCCI's disdain toward anti-doping regulations as designed by WADA is evident from its decision in the ADRV cases reported till date. One of the earliest cases of doping reported by BCCI, as evident from the ICC website, is that of Pradeep Sangwan.[190] Pradeep Sangwan tested positive for stanozolol.[191] It is an anabolic agent prohibited at all times as per the WADA list of Prohibited Substances/Methods.[192] The player did not deny the ADRV but pleaded that it was a case of inadvertent doping. He ingested the substance unknowingly with the medicines that he needed to take. That he was ignorant and innocent and came from a rural background.[193] The Tribunal analyzed the facts and found that the player was not aware of the anti-doping program as mandated by the WADA Code. That though the BCCI on paper has adopted the WADA Code 2009, it has been lax in conducting anti-doping education programs for the players. Consequently, the player having come from the rural background was ignorant of his duties under the anti-doping program. Further, the materials circulated among the players with regard to information on the anti-doping program were in English. The player was not conversant with English and hence could not follow the information given in the booklets. The Tribunal accepted the submission of the player that due to intake of medicines to burn his fat the prohibited substance entered his system. The Tribunal also accepted that

> the player's evidence that he believed, wrongly, that a product containing a banned substance would carry a warning to that effect on the packet. . . .

We accept also that he had no awareness of the risk that the fat burner tablets could contain a banned substance."[194]

Thus having accepted the innocence and ignorance of the player in the concerned matter, the Tribunal was to determine the ineligibility period. The Tribunal acknowledged that the conduct of the player cannot be regarded as a case of "No Fault or Negligence."[195] Accordingly, the Tribunal discussed the issue of the ineligibility period under the topic of No Significant Fault or Negligence.[196] Tribunal observed that the

> player submits that his fault was not significant because he lacked knowledge of prohibited substances; the ingestion was inadvertent; he was open about his use of the tablets; he promptly admitted the rule violation; he did not intend to enhance his performance. . . .[197]

The Tribunal accepted the argument given on behalf of the player that "antidoping education in Indian cricket has not yet permeated through to all players. We are conscious that in other sports such as international tennis, a high degree of personal anti-doping education is provided to each player."[198] Accordingly, the Tribunal held that the player's "ignorance of what substances are banned and what products may contain them, is to some extent excused by an absence of antidoping education and lack of fluent English."[199] Accordingly, the Tribunal held that "the player is able to show that his fault and negligence was not "significant." The player was at fault for trusting his gym instructor, but his fault was not significant when viewed in the totality of the circumstances."[200] The circumstances that convinced the Tribunal were that the "player was injured, that the fat burner tablets were taken out of competition, and that his motive was to lose weight rather than directly to enhance his performance."[201] However, the Tribunal ended up imposing ineligibility of 18 months on the ground that the player ought to have been more diligent in his conduct. Though the Tribunal backdated the starting date of the ineligibility significantly. Hence, though the decision was rendered on October 18, 2013, it was backdated to May 6, 2013. Accordingly, in effect, the player was to be ineligible for 12 months. This decision like the ones previously analyzed is flawed. To begin with, the substance for which the player was charged with ADRV is banned for all times as per the Prohibited List of WADA.[202] The holding of the Tribunal that since the out-of-competition ingestion of the substance proves No Significant Fault or Negligence is thus untenable. Second, the player at the time of the case was 22 years old and hence cannot be regarded as too young for the purpose of Article 10.5.2.[203] As per the commentary given therein, the defense of youth is applicable primarily in the case of a minor. Hence, the Tribunal's acceptance of the player's version as the correct explanation of the source of the substance is problematic. More so since there was no scientific proof to establish which of the medicines or fat burner tablets contained stanozolol. Finally, the holding of the Tribunal that the player blindly believing his gym instructor does not amount to significant fault is also not tenable. The Tribunal's assessment of the facts and arguments to hold No Significant Fault or Negligence is thus contrary to established CAS jurisprudence. For example, in *Alexandra Georgiana Radu v. Romanian National Anti-Doping Agency (RNADA)*, CAS reiterated that

> It is . . . irrelevant that an athlete allegedly did not receive any formal drug education from his/her club or federation prior to his/her first in-competition drug test as long as the athlete is found capable of understanding anti-doping requirements.[204]

Hence, an athlete by "having voluntarily and knowingly ingested pills, despite suspicions of their possibly performance enhancing effects . . . acted negligently and cannot establish a truly exceptional circumstance sufficient to reduce his/her negligence or the applicable standard sanction of 2 years."[205] Accordingly, the decision of the Tribunal herein does not satisfy the principles as laid by CAS.

The next reported case involves a charge of ADRV against Yusuf Pathan.[206] The substance found was terbutaline, a beta-2-agonists and prohibited at all times by WADA.[207] The player admitted to ADRV but contended that the substance was ingested by consuming the wrong medicine.[208] BCCI, in order to determine the period of ineligibility, assessed the facts as narrated by the player. Accordingly, BCCI accepted that the player had no intention to increase his performance.[209] That the ingestion of the prohibited substance was unwitting and accidental.[210] That the medicine consumed was prescribed by a doctor who was aware that the player was a cricketer.[211] That a trusted person was sent to get the medicine from the chemist.[212] And it was the medicine seller who gave the wrong medicine containing the prohibited substance.[213] The person in turn gave the medicine to the player who in good faith consumed the said medicine, days before his sample was collected for test. Hence, the player and the BCCI both relied on these facts to determine the degree of fault of the player. And it is not surprising to find that BCCI held, based on above-stated facts, that the player could prove No Significant Fault or Negligence.[214] This decision once again mocks at the efficacy of the entire anti-doping program. And it also deviates from the settled jurisprudence pertaining to the establishment of the degree of fault of the player.

In *Sara Errani v. International Tennis Federation (ITF)* and *National Anti-Doping Organisation (Nado) Italia v. Sara Errani and ITF*[215] for instance, CAS reiterated that "Athlete's responsibility includes that she is responsible for the behaviour of her entourage, be it her coaches, medical staff etc."[216] The player, as in this case, cannot give such a mundane excuse to reduce the ineligibility period. Importantly, the player cannot blame others for his/her negligence. It is also important to note that Article 10.5.1 of the 2015 WADA Code was applicable to this case.[217] According to CAS, by applying No Significant Fault or Negligence under Article 10.5.1 "a reduction can no longer be granted for the category of significant fault but only for a normal or light degree of fault or negligence."[218] In this case, the player's fault was definitely not normal or light. It was serious but BCCI imposed an ineligibility period of only 5 months. Further, BCCI backdated the starting of the ineligibility period resulting in the player effectively being ineligible for a week.[219] One cannot find a more ridiculous example of an ADRV decision than this. And it need not be re-stated that this is a clear example of BCCI's disregard of the WADA Code compliance requirement. In the Abhishek Gupta case, the charge of ADRV was based on the presence of a prohibited substance in the player's sample.[220] The substance was Terbutaline, a beta-2-agonists and prohibited at all times by WADA.[221] Here too, the BCCI gave the decision based on the admission of the player and his acceptance of the ADRV. Since the player did not challenge the finding of ADRV and had waived his right to a hearing, BCCI was not required to constitute a hearing panel.[222]

Surprisingly here too, the explanation given by the player for the ADRV is similar to the one given by Mr. Yusuf Pathan.[223] Accordingly here too, the player pleaded that the ADRV was inadvertent. The source of the substance was ingestion of a medication containing the prohibited substance. And the same was prescribed by the doctor.[224] And the medication was required because of cough and cold as well as throat infection that the player has developed.[225] Here, the medicine concerned has mentioned terbutaline sulphate as one of its ingredients on the label on the bottle.[226] Hence, ideally the player ought to have been cautious and refrained from using the same. However, BCCI does not regard this as a serious oversight on the part of the player. BCCI on the other notes that (a) the player did not consume the substance to enhance performance, (b) the player did not self-medicate and the medicine was prescribed by a qualified doctor, (c) the player declared voluntarily all the medicines he was taking, including the one containing terbutaline sulphate, (d) there was no performance-enhancing effect from the consumption of the medicine, and (e) he did not have any exposure to anti-doping education and level of awareness was inadequate.[227] These points persuaded BCCI to hold a finding in favor of No Significant Fault or Negligence. Importantly here, the BCCI applied the CAS jurisprudence on interpretation of Article 10.5.1.[228] And thus, the lapses on the part of the player were treated as normal fault or negligence.[229] Here too, BCCI could not stop itself from creating absurdity through its reasoning.

The BCCI compared the facts herein with those in the Yusuf Pathan case for the purpose of determining the period of ineligibility. It declared that the degree of fault of the player in the latter case was lesser. At the same time, it declared that the exposure level of Mr. Pathan was greater as compared to Mr. Gupta.[230] One wonders that with greater exposure and awareness how the degree of fault can be lesser. Importantly in Mr. Pathan's case, BCCI did not go into the interpretation of No Fault or Negligence, as laid down by CAS. Hence to make a statement without any substantive analysis takes away the merit from the BCCI decision. Proceeding with this analysis, the BCCI imposed an ineligibility period of 8 months on Mr. Gupta.[231] Here too, the sanction was imposed by backdating to the date of sample collection. In effect, the player ended up serving 4 months of ineligibility.[232] On July 30, 2019, BCCI gave a decision in ADRV cases involving three players. In the case of Akshay Dullarwar, the substance found was desacetyl deflazacort.[233] Desacetyl Deflazacort is a metabolite of Deflazacort and is a specified substance banned in-competition.[234] In this case, also the player promptly admitted the commission of the ADRV and pleaded his innocence.[235] The player explained the ADRV by pleading that it was accidental. It was caused by the consumption of tablets containing deflazacort. The said tablets were prescribed by the doctor for treating an infection. Further, he pleaded his ignorance and lack of anti-doping education as a ground to be considered by the BCCI. He also pleaded that his youth needs to be also taken into account.[236] Here too, the player waived his right to a hearing and accepted the decision of the BCCI. Accordingly, no Anti-Doping Panel was constituted for the same.[237]

In this case, also BCCI relied on the CAS jurisprudence pertaining to the interpretation of No Significant Fault or Negligence.[238] Accordingly, BCCI held that the player did not ingest the substance for enhancing performance. Neither did the player self-medicate nor did he hide information pertaining to the medicines he was using. Finally, the medicine had no performance-enhancing benefit insofar as the player is concerned.[239] BCCI also considered that the player was 22 years old and had less exposure to anti-doping education. Accordingly, an 8-month period of ineligibility was imposed on the player.[240] Here too, BCCI backdates the ineligibility period to the date of sample collection. Accordingly, the player effectively is required to serve 4 months of ineligibility.[241] In the second case of the same date, Mr. Divya Gajraj was charged with ADRV for a prohibited substance.[242] However, unlike all the cases discussed so far, this involved a minor. The player was, at the time of the finding of ADRV, 17 years of age.[243] The substance found in his sample was acetazolamide.[244] It is prohibited at all times and is a specified substance under the WADA Prohibited List.[245] Here too, the player accepted ADRV and explained it as inadvertent doping. The same having been caused by ingestion of medicine containing the prohibited substance. The said medicine was prescribed by a doctor.[246] Like in the previous case, here too the player waive his right to a hearing and accepted the decision of BCCI. Consequently here too, no Panel was constituted by the BCCI.[247] And here, the player justifiably pleaded his youth and limited anti-doping education as a ground to reduce the ineligibility period.[248]

Here too BCCI, like in the previous cases, considered the fact that the player had not intended to increase the performance nor did he self-medicate, and there was no performance-enhancing effect of the medicine.[249] However, the one thing that is different in the given facts is that the player failed to disclose the medicine he was using.[250] However, the BCCI did not regard that as an important omission. Accordingly, the BCCI considered the fault of the player as normal especially taking into account his youth and poor anti-doping education.[251] Accordingly, BCCI applied its discretion and imposed an ineligibility period of 6 months. The same was, however, backdated as a result the player had to serve an ineligibility period of 3 months only.[252] The last case of ADRV as decided by BCCI on that day involved Mr. Prithvi Shaw.[253] The player, at the time of the ADRV, was 19 years old. His sample tested positive for terbutaline, a beta-2-agonists, which was prohibited at all times by WADA.[254] He too, like the others, accepted the ADRV without protest and pleaded that it was inadvertent. He explained that the source of the prohibited substance was a medicine which he was prescribed by the pharmacist. The medicine was needed to treat his condition of cough and cold. He further pleaded his youth and lack of experience as well as his career opportunities likely to be affected by the ADRV. He pleaded that BCCI should consider all the above reasons to reduce his potential period of ineligibility.[255]

The player herein also accepts the decision of the BCCI and waives his right to hearing. Hence as in the previous cases, the BCCI is not required to constitute a panel.[256] A thing that is unique about this case, as against the other two cases, is the status of the player. Despite his youth, the player is an international level player. He has been a member of the Indian National Team and represented India in both Test matches and One Day Internationals.[257] Importantly, the player was selected for the Australian tour, which he missed because of injury. Consequently, he returned to India, and it is here that while recovering from the injury, the player suffered from cough and cold. He consulted his father who suggested a visit to the local pharmacy for getting medicine for the cough and cold. Accordingly, the player visited the pharmacy and bought an over-the-counter syrup to treat his cough and cold. It is also relevant that the player did not bother to consult a specialist for the medicine nor did he make attempt to find out the ingredients of the syrup. He, being an international level player, was comparatively lax in his approach to the use of the medicine. He confessed that he does not remember the name of the medicine. However, he alleged, without any scientific evidence, that such medicines do contain the prohibited substance.[258] BCCI, however, does not have any problem in accepting this version of the player. It does not look for scientific evidence. It does not refer to the fact that the player, while filling up the doping control form, failed to mention the details of the syrup consumed.[259] BCCI accepts calmly that the syrup was the source of the prohibited substance.[260] The BCCI states that

> irrespective of what Mr Shaw should have been thinking in respect of his use of medication, the BCCI accepts his assertion that he took the cough syrup merely to alleviate his symptoms, and not with the intent to enhance (or with the effect of enhancing) his sports performance."[261]

Having thus set the tone of the findings, the next step for the BCCI was to determine the period of ineligibility to be imposed. Considering that the BCCI was convinced about the innocence of the player, his conduct too received a sympathetic assessment. Accordingly, BCCI holds that the player did not ingest the prohibited substance to enhance performance. He used it to cure his cough and cold. BCCI further holds that the player did not self-medicate because the medicine was given to him by a pharmacist. This assessment of the BCCI is amazing considering that when over-the-counter medicines are bought without consulting a doctor, it is a case of self-medication. Hilariously, BCCI notes that the player could be excused for believing that the over-the-counter medicine will have no prohibited substance. Finally, the BCCI concluded that the medicine does not appear to have had any performance-enhancing effect on the player.[262] Consequently, the BCCI considered the case as that of a normal fault. And hence, the player was regarded as having committed No Significant Fault or Negligence. The BCCI reiterated that in arriving at this conclusion the player's youth, inexperience, lack of anti-doping education as well as his anxiety to get back to form have been considered.[263] Accordingly, BCCI imposed an ineligibility period of 8 months which was backdated to the date of sample collection. Consequently, the player was required to serve an ineligibility period of 4 months.[264] This thus concludes the review of the decisions as reported on the ICC website and decided by the BCCI. These decisions do not inspire confidence that the BCCI will change its track post-August 2019.

As the cases reveal, BCCI never denied that it is against the WADA Code. Neither could it so deny considering that it is under the jurisdiction of ICC. Hence, at least on paper, the BCCI along with the ICC continued with their lip service toward compliance requirement.[265] As the cases indicate, BCCI in almost all of them did refer to the anti-doping jurisprudence developed by CAS. BCCI, while rendering a decision, did invoke the principles as developed by CAS. BCCI did refer to the WADA Code while deciding the matters of ADRV. Unfortunately, though the implementation leaves a lot to be desired, BCCI with its power play in the field of cricket cannot be compelled by the ICC to be WADA Code compliant. Further, as noted earlier, ICC needs BCCI to sustain the game and generate revenue. Hence, ICC and BCCI have to bear each other with a lot of adjustments and compromise. In all this, ICC can easily be hauled up by both the IOC and WADA for its failure to ensure BCCI's compliance. Article 12 of the WADA Code 2021 clearly lays down that the Signatories will ensure that their members comply with the requirements of the WADA Code.[266] In addition to this WADA Code 2021 also imposes further compliance obligations on the IFs. As per Article 20.3.2, the IFs are to ensure that membership is only granted to National Federations that strictly comply with the WADA Code.[267] ICC fails on both counts as it has till date not taken any action against BCCI for failing in WADA Code compliance. The other problem with the decisions given by BCCI is that they lack substantial reasons to justify the outcome.

Hence, the variance in the period of punishment for similar ADRVs is not comprehendible. Further, it is problematic for BCCI to be the prosecutor as well as the adjudicator. It is the one who frames the charges, and it is the one who decides the case. It, therefore, is not surprising that the players, in most cases of ADRV, have accepted the decision of the BCCI. For there is clearly an inequality of bargaining power. The players are being adjudicated by the body which also is responsible for their playing career. BCCI determines the issue of selection as well as other related aspects of a player's career. Hence, it is always beneficial for the players to enter into a compromise with the BCCI and hope for leniency. This form of justice delivery system also goes against the requirement of compliance. For the players are thus manipulated into admission as well as the ADRV is dealt with more leniently. The understanding between the BCCI and player seems to be that BCCI will ensure the players' are let off with a lighter punishment. And the players will accept whatever findings BCCI gives. This affects both the innocent and the guilty. For the innocent gets punished without having done the wrong and the guilty get released after serving a lesser quantum of ineligibility period. The BCCI thus has absolute control over the players in terms of what they can or they cannot do. Hence, BCCI can at its whims and fancy allow the players to use performance-enhancing drugs and not get caught. BCCI, by being the sole adjudicator of the offense, is also running an opaque system. It does not have any system through which players are allowed access to an independent body for adjudication.

It was these considerations that led the Government of India to put pressure on BCCI and force it to accept NADA.[268] One can have a lot of things to say about NADA[269] but the point remains that it is independent of BCCI. Hence in terms of ensuring fairness in the procedure of adjudication, the BCCI and players both will be equally placed. Further, the players will be in a better position to contest the finding of ADRV. The players will be in a better position to argue their case. The players will be in a better position to defend their rights.[270] ICC too can breathe easy for the acceptance of NADA is a positive step toward WADA Code compliance on its part. ICC can now claim to have discharged its burden of ensuring that BCCI is in compliance with the WADA Code.[271] NADA being recognized by WADA,[272] BCCI's acceptance of NADA is a positive step. However, as mentioned earlier, time will prove whether acceptance of NADA indeed is fruitful. For the power equation between BCCI and other NCFs remains unchanged. BCCI is the boss of the cricket world and the other NCFs cannot complain about the same. The ICC too cannot complain against the BCCI for it too is dependent on BCCI for revenue generation. As the National Federation of the most popular sport in the second-most populous country automatically spells money and power. The only entities which can have any say in the matter will be IOC and WADA. For their clout and power are equal to BCCI. They can continue to effectively monitor the compliance of ICC as well as nudge ICC to ensure compliance of BCCI.

Conclusion

The South Asian market of cricket is too big to be ignored and ICC realizes the same. Further IPL has changed the narrative to an extent that it rivals all official matches in terms of popularity. Given this scenario, the acceptance of NADA by BCCI is indeed a great achievement for all concerned. However, one has to be skeptical about the fruitfulness of this development. A cursory look through BCCI's website does not reveal much. Importantly, the link to NADA has not yet been updated. It continues to take one to the 2015 WADA Code, as adopted by NADA. On the other hand, NADA has updated its Code version as well the Prohibited list. The same is in compliance with the 2021 version. Further unlike the ICC website, BCCI does not have any information about the whereabouts filing or its procedure, as designed for the players. Importantly, there is no information that a person will get from the BCCI's webpage on Anti-Doping. It is as sparse as it can be and gives minimal information on the steps BCCI has taken or will take to ramp up the anti-doping measures. Insofar as ICC is concerned, its hand are clearly tied due to the financial incentive that BCCI provides. While on paper, ICC appears to be taking steps for effective compliance the same falls short of expected standards. And, ICC's dilemma vis-à-vis BCCI is also reflective of the privilege that the Non-Olympic sport enjoys when it comes to WADA Code compliance. Hence, neither ICC nor BCCI is likely to face the heat from IOC or WADA for its poor record. And the fact that IOC continues to recognize ICC despite all the laxity on the part of its member NCF is revealing. The IOC too can wield the stick only if the sport is part of the Olympic program. And the ICC BCCI tussle exemplifies this as it has been seen in the case of IFAF and NFL. And this inherent dichotomy between Olympic and Non-Olympic sports vis-à-vis the anti-doping compliance continues to challenge the legitimacy of the WADA Code.

Notes

1. PTI, "IOC Recognizes ICC, Cricket Can Now Become Olympic Sport" www. livemint.com/Consumer/C6ANnHs0Zbme94bLoZOf5O/IOC-recognizes-ICC-cricket-can-now-become-Olympic-sport.html (accessed 20th February 2021)
2. ARISF, "Members" www.arisf.sport/members.aspx (accessed 20th February 2021)
3. ICC Anti-Doping, "ICC Anti-Doping Code" www.icc-cricket.com/about/integrity/anti-doping/code (accessed 20th February 2021)
4. Ibid
5. World Anti-Doping Agency, "World Anti-Doping Code 2021" www.wada-ama.org/sites/default/files/resources/files/2021_wada_code.pdf (accessed 21 February 2021)
6. ICC Anti-Doping (n 3), Article 1
7. Ibid Article 2
8. Ibid Article 3
9. World Anti-Doping Agency (n 5) [Article 23.2.-Implementation of the Code]
10. International Cricket Council, "Player's Consent and Agreement to the ICC Anti-Doping Code" https://icc-static-files.s3.amazonaws.com/ICC/document/2019/05/02/de344f3b-1ba1-4a67-b5a8-745172f7e826/ICC-Player-s-Consent-and-Agreement-form.pdf (accessed 20th February 2021)
11. Ibid
12. International Cricket Council (n 10)
13. Ibid
14. "National Cricket Federations Anti-Doping Rules Template Effective 1 January 2021" https://resources.pulse.icc-cricket.com/ICC/document/2021/01/14/c52a3589-f99d-4d5b-a078-ec97f90ce1fe/National-Cricket-Federations-Anti-Doping-Rules-Template-effective-1Jan21.pdf (accessed 20th February 2021)

15. International Cricket Council (n 3) "Whereabouts Requirements for Out-of Competition Testing- Effective Date, 1 January 2021" https://resources.pulse.icc-cricket.com/ICC/document/2020/12/31/de7262c0-b6d9-4550-a2a6-ca85700292e2/Whereabouts-Regulations-effective-1-Jan-2021.pdf (accessed 20th February 2021)

16. World Anti-Doping Agency, "The World Anti-Doping Code International Standard Testing and Investigations" www.wada-ama.org/sites/default/files/resources/files/international_standard_isti_-_2020.pdf (accessed 20th February 2021)

17. Ibid

18. Ibid

19. Ibid

20. International Cricket Council, "About Our Members" [Full Members are the governing bodies for cricket of a country recognised by the ICC, or nations associated for cricket purposes, or a geographical area, from which representative teams are qualified to play official Test matches (12 Members).] www.icc-cricket.com/about/members/about-our-members (accessed 20th February 2021)

21. Ibid

22. Ibid [2B. Whereabouts requirements for National Cricket Federations in the NCFP-2.3 National Cricket Federations included in the NCFP are required to submit two sets of whereabouts information to the ICC. Whereabouts information relating to its national representative teams participating in International Matches and whereabouts information relating to Specified Domestic Events taking place under its jurisdiction, in both cases as more particularly described below. (i) International Matches 2.4 National Cricket Federations in the NCFP are responsible for providing the ICC, through ADAMS, with full details (location, full address, dates, times, overnight accommodation) for all days when its senior national representative teams (including explicitly any NPP Players) will be together for the purposes of training for or playing in International Matches (irrespective of what format of cricket such representative team may be playing) as well as the date(s) and full address of each place the Players in the national representatives teams will be staying overnight with the said team ("NCF International Team Filing). Alongside the NCF International Team Filing, the National Cricket Federation shall file with the ICC (via e-mail) a list of the names of all squad members involved in the International Matches to which the NCF International Team Filing relates, highlighting any NPP Player. For the avoidance of doubt, information relating to women's national representative teams is only required for those National Cricket Federations ranked in the top ten of the ICC Women's ODI Rankings.]

23. International Cricket Council (n 20).

24. Ibid [On or before 31 January in each calendar year, the ICC shall identify (at its sole discretion and save in exceptional circumstances), no more than one men's and one women's Specified Domestic Event per National Cricket Federation included in the NCFP for which the relevant National Cricket Federation shall be required to provide whereabouts information to the ICC in respect of such Specified Domestic Event. This requirement is in addition to the requirement to provide whereabouts information in respect of national representative teams as set out in Article 2.4 above. In circumstances where, after the ICC has designated a domestic league as a Specified Domestic Event, the name or format of the particular Specified Domestic Event changes, or is replaced by a different domestic league, the ICC shall be entitled (again at its sole discretion) to replace the existing identified domestic league with the new or amended league as the National Cricket Federation's Specified Domestic Event for that year.]

25. Ibid [No later than 14 days prior to the first scheduled match in the relevant Specified Domestic Event, the National Cricket Federation under whose jurisdiction the Specified Domestic Event is taking place must (to the best of its knowledge)

provide the ICC (via e-mail) with full details of the match and training schedule for the Specified Domestic Event (including, the dates and times of each team's training sessions and matches, the locations of each training session and match, as well as details of the team's overnight accommodation) (the "NCF Domestic Event Filing"). The NCF Domestic Event Filing shall also include a list of the names of all squad members in the team (in so far as such information is known at the date of submission), highlighting any NPP Player. If this information changes in the lead up to the Specified Domestic Event, the relevant National Cricket Federation shall update its NCF Domestic Event Filing accordingly. A failure by the National Cricket Federation to file the NCF Domestic Event Filing within the required deadline or to file complete information as set out above amounts to an NCF Filing Failure for the purposes of Article 2.8.]

26. Ibid [Article 2.9]
27. Ibid [Article 2.9.4]
28. Ibid [Article 2.9.3]
29. Ibid [Article 2.10]
30. International Cricket Council (n 20) Article 3
31. Ibid Article 3.4.1
32. Ibid Article 3.4.2
33. Ibid Article 3.4.3
34. Ibid
35. Ibid Article 3.10.1
36. Ibid Article 3.10.5
37. Ibid
38. Ibid Article 3.13
39. Ibid Article 4.5
40. International Cricket Council (n 20) Article 4.8 [Article 4.8.1 Each Player in the IRTP remains ultimately responsible at all times for making accurate and complete Whereabouts Filings in accordance with Article 4.5, whether he/she makes each filing personally or delegates it to a third party (or a mixture of the two). It will not be a defence to an allegation of a Filing Failure under ICC Code Article 2.4 that the Player delegated such responsibility to a third party and that third party failed to comply with the applicable requirements. 4.8.2 Such Player remains ultimately responsible at all times for ensuring he/she is available for Testing at the whereabouts declared on his/her Whereabouts Filings, whether he/she made that filing personally or delegated it to a third party (or a mixture of the two). It will not be a defence to an allegation of a Missed Test under ICC Code Article 2.4 that the Player delegated responsibility for filing his/her whereabouts information for the relevant period to a third party and that third party failed to comply with the applicable requirements.]
41. Ibid Article 4.15
42. ICC Anti-Doping (n 3)
43. World Anti-Doping Agency, "International Standards" [The World Anti-Doping Code (Code) is the core document that harmonizes anti-doping policies, rules and regulations within sport organizations and among public authorities around the world. It works in conjunction with the following eight International Standards that aim to foster consistency among anti-doping organizations in various areas: 1. Prohibited List 2. Testing and investigations. 3. Laboratories 4. Therapeutic Use Exemptions (TUEs) 5. Protection of Privacy and Personal Information 6. Code Compliance by Signatories 7. Education 8. Results Management. These International Standards have been the subject of lengthy consultation processes with WADA's stakeholders and are mandatory for all Signatories of the Code.] www.wada-ama.org/en/what-we-do/international-standards (accessed 21st February 2021)

44. ICC Anti-Doping (n 3)
45. World Anti-Doping Agency, "Athletes' Anti-Doping Rights Act- [Approved by WADA's Executive Committee on 7 November 2019.]" www.wada-ama.org/sites/default/files/resources/files/athlete_act_en.pdf (accessed 21st February 2021)
46. Ibid
47. Ibid
48. World Anti-Doping Agency (n 45)
49. Ibid
50. Ibid
51. ICC Anti-Doping, "Decisions and Periods of Ineligibility" www.icc-cricket.com/about/integrity/anti-doping/decisions-and-integrity (accessed 21st February 2021)
52. Chinmay Jawalekar, "Upul Tharanga: 11 Facts About the Consistently Inconsistent Sri Lankan Batsman" www.cricketcountry.com/articles/upul-tharanga-11-facts-about-the-consistently-inconsistent-sri-lankan-batsman-512257 (accessed 21st February 2021)
53. Cricbuzz, "Upul Tharanga Sri Lanka" www.cricbuzz.com/profiles/414/upul-tharanga#!#profile (accessed 21st February 2021)
54. "International Cricket Council Independent Anti-Doping Tribunal Decision in the Case of Mr Upul Tharanga" para 3 https://fdocuments.in/reader/full/international-cricket-council-independent-anti-doping (accessed 21st February 2021)
55. Ibid
56. World-Anti Doping Agency, "What Is Prohibited- Prohibited in-Competition" www.wada-ama.org/en/content/what-is-prohibited/prohibited-in-competition/glucocorticoids (accessed 21st February 2021)
57. International Cricket Council Independent Anti-Doping Tribunal Decision (n 54)
58. Ibid para 5
59. Ibid
60. Ibid
61. Ibid
62. Ibid para 6
63. World Anti-Doping Agency, "World Anti-Doping Code-2009" [10.2 Ineligibility for Presence, Use or Attempted Use, or Possession of Prohibited Substances and Prohibited Methods The period of Ineligibility imposed for a violation of Article 2.1 (Presence of Prohibited Substance or its Metabolites or Markers), Article 2.2 (Use or Attempted Use of Prohibited Substance or Prohibited Method) or Article 2.6 (Possession of Prohibited Substances and Prohibited Methods) shall be as follows, unless the conditions for eliminating or reducing the period of Ineligibility, as provided in Articles 10.4 and 10.5, or the conditions for increasing the period of Ineligibility, as provided in Article 10.6, are met: First violation: Two (2) years Ineligibility] www.wada-ama.org/sites/default/files/resources/files/wada_anti-doping_code_2009_en_0.pdf (accessed 21st February 2021)
64. Ibid [10.4 Elimination or Reduction of the Period of Ineligibility for Specified Substances under Specific Circumstances Where an Athlete or other Person can establish how a Specified Substance entered his or her body or came into his or her Possession and that such Specified Substance was not intended to enhance the Athlete's sport performance or mask the Use of a performance-enhancing substance, the period of Ineligibility found in Article 10.2 shall be replaced with the following: First violation: At a minimum, a reprimand and no period of Ineligibility from future Events, and at a maximum, two (2) years of Ineligibility. To justify any elimination or reduction, the Athlete or other Person must produce corroborating evidence in addition to his or her word which establishes to the comfortable satisfaction of the hearing panel the absence of an intent to enhance sport performance or mask the Use of a performance-enhancing substance. The Athlete's or other

Person's degree of fault shall be the criterion considered in assessing any reduction of the period of Ineligibility.]

65. World Anti-Doping Agency (n 62) [Comment to Article 10.4: Specified Substances are not necessarily less serious agents for purposes of sports doping than other Prohibited Substances (for example, a stimulant that is listed as a Specified Substance could be very effective to an Athlete in competition); for that reason, an Athlete who does not meet the criteria under this Article would receive a two-year period of Ineligibility and could receive up to a four-year period of Ineligibility under Article 10.6. However, there is a greater likelihood that Specified Substances, as opposed to other Prohibited Substances, could be susceptible to a credible, non-doping explanation. This Article applies only in those cases where the hearing panel is comfortably satisfied by the objective circumstances of the case that the Athlete in taking or Possessing a Prohibited Substance did not intend to enhance his or her sport performance. Examples of the type of objective circumstances which in combination might lead a hearing panel to be comfortably satisfied of no performance-enhancing intent would include: the fact that the nature of the Specified Substance or the timing of its ingestion would not have been beneficial to the Athlete; the Athlete's open Use or disclosure of his or her Use of the Specified Substance; and a contemporaneous medical records file substantiating the non-sport-related prescription for the Specified Substance. Generally, the greater the potential performance-enhancing benefit, the higher the burden on the Athlete to prove lack of an intent to enhance sport performance. While the absence of intent to enhance sport performance must be established to the comfortable satisfaction of the hearing panel, the Athlete may establish how the Specified Substance entered the body by a balance of probability. In assessing the Athlete's or other Person's degree of fault, the circumstances considered must be specific and relevant to explain the Athlete's or other Person's departure from the expected standard of behavior. Thus, for example, the fact that an Athlete would lose the opportunity to earn large sums of money during a period of Ineligibility or the fact that the Athlete only has a short time left in his or her career or the timing of the sporting calendar would not be relevant factors to be considered in reducing the period of Ineligibility under this Article. It is anticipated that the period of Ineligibility will be eliminated entirely in only the most exceptional cases]
66. International Cricket Council Independent Anti-Doping Tribunal (n 54)
67. Ibid para 15
68. Ibid para 21
69. Ibid para 30
70. Ibid para 37
71. Ibid para 39
72. International Cricket Council Independent Anti-Doping Tribunal (n 54) para 41
73. Ibid para 80
74. World Anti-Doping Agency (n 63)
75. International Cricket Council Independent Anti-Doping Tribunal (n 54) para 78
76. Ibid para 79
77. Ibid para 96
78. Ibid para 104
79. World Anti-Doping Agency (n 63)
80. CAS 2011/A/2515
81. Ibid para 27
82. Ibid para 9
83. Ibid para 7
84. Ibid para 8
85. Ibid para 30 [FINA Doping Control Rules had incorporated the WADA 2009 Code]

86. Ibid para 3
87. Ibid para 32
88. Ibid para 11
89. Ibid para 31
90. Ibid para 32
91. Ibid para 70
92. Ibid para 75
93. Ibid para 77
94. ESPNcricinfo Staff, "Treymane Smartt Suspended for Anti-Doping Violation" www.espncricinfo.com/story/west-indies-news-treymane-smartt-suspended-for-anti-doping-violation-541123 (accessed 21st February 2021)
95. Ibid
96. World-AntiDopingAgency, "ProhibitedatAllTimes-DiureticsandMaskingAgents" www.wada-ama.org/en/content/what-is-prohibited/prohibited-at-all-times/diuretics-and-masking-agents (accessed 21st February 2021)
97. ESPNcricinfo Staff (n 94)
98. Ibid
99. "International Cricket Council and Yasir Shah Disciplinary Proceedings Under the ICC Anti-Doping Code 2015" http://icc-live.s3.amazonaws.com/cms/media/about_docs/56c837d5b5413-Yasir%20Shah%20-%20Agreed%20Decision%20FINAL%2007%20February%202016%20WEBSITE.PDF (accessed 21st February 2021)
100. World-Anti Doping Agency (n 96)
101. "Significant Changes between the 2009 Code and the 2015 Code, Version 4.0" www.wada-ama.org/sites/default/files/wadc-2015-draft-version-4.0-significant-changes-to-2009-en.pdf (accessed 22nd February 2021)
102. International Cricket Council (n 99) para 26
103. World-Anti Doping Agency, "World Anti-Doping Code 2015" [10.5.1 Reduction of Sanctions for Specified Substances or Contaminated Products for Violations of Article 2.1, 2.2 or 2.6–10.5.1.1 Specified Substances-Where the anti-doping rule violation involves a Specified Substance, and the Athlete or other Person can establish No Significant Fault or Negligence, then the period of Ineligibility shall be, at a minimum, a reprimand and no period of Ineligibility, and at a maximum, two years of Ineligibility, depending on the Athlete's or other Person's degree of Fault.] www.wada-ama.org/sites/default/files/resources/files/wada-2015-world-anti-doping-code.pdf (accessed 22nd February 2021)
104. International Cricket Council (n 99) para 28
105. Ibid para 29
106. World-Anti Doping Agency, "Prohibited List Q&A" www.wada-ama.org/en/questions-answers/prohibited-list-qa (accessed 22nd February 2021)
107. International Cricket Council (n 99) para 27
108. Ibid para 28
109. World-Anti Doping Agency (n 103) [10.5.2 Application of No Significant Fault or Negligence beyond the Application of Article 10.5.1- If an Athlete or other Person establishes in an individual case where Article 10.5.1 is not applicable, that he or she bears No Significant Fault or Negligence, then, subject to further reduction or elimination as provided in Article 10.6, the otherwise applicable period of Ineligibility may be reduced based on the Athlete or other Person's degree of Fault, but the reduced period of Ineligibility may not be less than one-half of the period of Ineligibility otherwise applicable. If the otherwise applicable period of Ineligibility is a lifetime, the reduced period under this Article may be no less than eight years.]
110. International Cricket Council (n 99) para 29

111. International Cricket Council (n 20)

112. "In the Matter of Proceedings brought Under the BCB Anti-Doping Rules Between: The Bangladesh Cricket Board and Mr Kaz!Anik Islam" https://resources.pulse. icc-cricket.com/ICC/document/2020/07/27/764211fb-135d-4089-aa55-debd d1080eb3/Kazi-Anik-AD-decision.pdf (accessed 22nd February 2021)

113. World-Anti Doping Agency, "World Anti-Doping Code International Standard Prohibited List" www.wada-ama.org/sites/default/files/resources/files/2021list_ en.pdf (accessed 22nd February 2021)

114. World-Anti Doping Agency (n 103) [2.1 Presence of a Prohibited Substance or its Metabolites or Markers in an Athlete's Sample]

115. Ibid [2.1.2 Sufficient proof of an anti-doping rule violation under Article 2.1 is established by any of the following: presence of a Prohibited Substance or its Metabolites or Markers in the Athlete's A Sample where the Athlete waives analysis of the B Sample and the B Sample is not analyzed; or, where the Athlete's B Sample is analyzed and the analysis of the Athlete's B Sample confirms the presence of the Prohibited Substance or its Metabolites or Markers found in the Athlete's A Sample; or, where the Athlete's B Sample is split into two bottles and the analysis of the second bottle confirms the presence of the Prohibited Substance or its Metabolites or Markers found in the first bottle]

116. In the Matter of (n 112) para 12–13

117. World-Anti Doping Agency (n 103) [Article 10.6.3 Prompt Admission of an Anti-Doping Rule Violation after being Confronted with a Violation Sanctionable under Article 10.2.1 or Article 10.3.1 An Athlete or other Person potentially subject to a four-year sanction under Article 10.2.1 or 10.3.1 (for evading or refusing Sample Collection or Tampering with Sample Collection), by promptly admitting the asserted anti-doping rule violation after being confronted by an Anti-Doping Organization, and also upon the approval and at the discretion of both WADA and the Anti-Doping Organization with results management responsibility, may receive a reduction in the period of Ineligibility down to a minimum of two years, depending on the seriousness of the violation and the Athlete or other Person's degree of Fault.]

118. In the Matter of (n 112) para 18

119. World-Anti Doping Agency (n 103) [10.2.1 The period of Ineligibility shall be four years where: 10.2.1.1 The anti-doping rule violation does not involve a Specified Substance. . .]

120. In the Matter of (n 112) para 20

121. Ibid para 22–23

122. Ibid para 24

123. "Before the Sports Tribunal of New Zealand-Drug Free Sport New Zealand and Harrisyn Jones and New Zealand Cricket" https://icc-static-files.s3.amazonaws. com/ICC/document/2018/09/20/b3f51e27-455a-40d0-824c-7cdebc2b23b7/ ST0518-Decision.pdf (accessed 22nd February 2021)

124. World-Anti Doping Agency (n 106)

125. Before the Sports Tribunal (n 123) para 10

126. "The Anti-Doping Tribunal-in the Adjudication Proceeding Between Pakistan Cricket Board (PCB) and Kashif Saddique" http://icc-live.s3.amazonaws.com/ cms/media/about_docs/537498900afda-PCB%20-%20Kashif%20Siddique%20 -%20Apr%202014.pdf (accessed 22nd February 2021)

127. World-Anti Doping Agency, "Prohibited at All Times" www.wada-ama.org/ en/content/what-is-prohibited/prohibited-at-all-times/anabolic-agents (accessed 22nd February 2021)

128. The Anti-Doping Tribunal (n 126) para 26

129. Ibid para 28

130. Ibid para 33–34
131. Ibid para 36
132. World-Anti Doping Agency (n 63)
133. The Anti-Doping Tribunal (n 126) para 40
134. "In the Matter of Raza Hasan, Cricketer" http://icc-live.s3.amazonaws.com/cms/media/about_docs/556ab7b724b5d-In%20the%20Matter%20of%20Raza%20Hasan%20(Cricketer).pdf (accessed 22nd February 2021)
135. Ibid para 4
136. World-Anti Doping Agency, "Substances of Abuse Under the 2021 World Anti-Doping Code Guidance Note for Anti-Doping Organizations" www.wada-ama.org/sites/default/files/resources/files/2020-01-11_guidance_note_on_substances_of_abuse_en_0.pdf (accessed 22nd February 2021); The World Anti-Doping Code, "The 2015 Prohibited List International Standard" www.wada-ama.org/sites/default/files/resources/files/wada-2015-prohibited-list-en.pdf (accessed 22nd February 2021)
137. In the Matter of Raza Hasan (n 134) para 8
138. Ibid para 9–10
139. Ibid para 12
140. World-Anti Doping Agency (n 63)
141. World-Anti Doping Agency (n 103) [Article 10.2.1 The period of Ineligibility shall be four years where: 10.2.1.1 The anti-doping rule violation does not involve a Specified Substance, unless the Athlete or other Person can establish that the anti-doping rule violation was not intentional.]
142. ESPNcricinfo Staff, "Rehman Banned for 12 Weeks for Cannabis Use" www.espncricinfo.com/story/abdur-rehman-banned-for-12-weeks-for-cannabis-585337 (accessed 22nd February 2021)
143. The World Anti-Doping Code, "The 2012 Prohibited List International Standard" www.wada-ama.org/sites/default/files/resources/files/WADA_Prohibited_List_2012_EN.pdf (accessed 22nd February 2021)
144. World-Anti Doping Agency (n 63)
145. ESPNcricinfo Staff (n 142)
146. World-Anti Doping Agency (n 63)
147. "SA Institute for Drug Free Sport (SAIDS) Anti Doping Disciplinary Hearing: Mr Rory Kleinveldt and Cricket South Africa ("CSA")" www.doping.nl/media/kb/1439/SAIDS%20Kleinveldt%202012-07%20(S).pdf (accessed 22nd February 2021)
148. The World Anti-Doping Code (n 143)
149. World-Anti Doping Agency (n 63)
150. Ibid
151. SA Institute for Drug Free Sport (SAIDS) (n 147)
152. Ibid
153. Ibid
154. Ibid
155. SA Institute for Drug Free Sport (SAIDS) (n 147)
156. "The Jamaica Anti-Doping Disciplinary Panel Between Jamaica Anti-Doping Commission and Odean Brown" http://icc-live.s3.amazonaws.com/cms/media/about_docs/578612fba01e6-OdeanBrown.pdf (accessed 22nd February 2021)
157. Ibid para 95
158. Ibid para 99
159. World-Anti Doping Agency (n 103) [For violations of Article 2.4, the period of Ineligibility shall be two years, subject to reduction down to a minimum of one year, depending on the Athlete's degree of Fault. The flexibility between two years and one year of Ineligibility in this Article is not available to Athletes where

a pattern of last-minute whereabouts changes or other conduct raises a serious suspicion that the Athlete was trying to avoid being available for Testing.]

160. Ibid
161. The Jamaica Anti-Doping Disciplinary (n 156) para 143–144
162. Ibid para 141
163. BCCI, "About the BCCI" www.bcci.tv/about/history (accessed 23rd February 2021)
164. Sportskeeda, "For Cricket to Grow Globally, BCCI's Power Needs to Be Curtailed: Part 1" https://cricket.yahoo.net/news/for-cricket-grow-globally-bcci-s-power-needs-curtailed-part-1 (accessed 23rd February 2021)
165. Shamik Chakrabarty, "India Is a Global Power in Cricket . . . Position Cannot Be Compromised: BCCI Secretary Ajay Shirke" https://indianexpress.com/article/sports/cricket/india-global-power-cricket-position-cannot-compromised-bcci-secretary-ajay-shirke-3023340/ (accessed 23rd February 2021)
166. Aswathi R. Jayachandran, "BCCI-ICC: The Tug of Financial War" https://medium.com/crimpulse/bcci-icc-the-tug-of-financial-war-fddf2a540696 (accessed 23rd February 2021)
167. Team Bridge, "In India Cricket Is a Religion, as Football Is in European Countries" https://thebridge.in/latest/india-cricket-religion-football-in-european-countries/#:~:text=Mecca%20of%20making%20money!&text=Thus%2C%20cricket%20is%20not%20only,has%20generated%20loads%20of%20revenue. (accessed 23rd February 2021)
168. Worldometer, "India Population" www.worldometers.info/world-population/india-population/ (accessed 23rd February 2021)
169. Martin Williamson, "How the World Cup Became a Commercial Hit" www.espncricinfo.com/story/martin-williamson-how-the-world-cup-became-a-commercial-hit-824079 (accessed 23rd February 2021)
170. https://twitter.com/mohanstatsman/status/981897579226165248 (accessed 23rd February 2021)
171. Ashish Magotra, "From 1983's Miracle Win to Financial Might of IPL: How India Increased Control Over World Cricket" https://scroll.in/field/958713/from-1983s-miracle-win-to-financial-might-of-ipl-how-india-increased-control-over-world-cricket (accessed 23rd February 2021)
172. Venkat Ananth, "How BCCI Became the 800-Pound Gorilla of Cricket" www.livemint.com/Consumer/pVdCJRSBBid7eVxuCwfqcK/How-India-became-the-800-pound-gorilla-of-cricket.html (accessed 23rd February 2021)
173. Sharda Ugra, "Match Referee Mike Denness' Harsh Sentences Pitch BCCI into Confrontation with ICC" www.indiatoday.in/magazine/cover-story/story/20011203-match-referee-mike-denness-harsh-sentences-pitch-bcci-into-confrontation-with-icc-774971-2001-12-03 (accessed 23rd February 2021)
174. Martin Williamson, "The Denness Affair" www.espncricinfo.com/magazine/content/story/496743.html (accessed 23rd February 2021)
175. V.S. Aravind, "Denness the Menace- When Tendulkar Was Called 'Cheat'" www.sify.com/sports/denness-the-menace--when-tendulkar-was-called-cheat-news-cricket-pj2qbrhddgjfb.html (accessed 23rd February 2021)
176. Aabhas Sharma, "Jagmohan Dalmiya: The Man Who Showed Who Is the Boss" www.rediff.com/cricket/report/jagmohan-dalmiya-the-man-who-showed-who-is-the-boss-bcci-sachin-tendulkar-ball-tampering-pix/20150922.htm (accessed 23rd February 2021)
177. Arunabha Sengupta, "Mike Denness: English Captain Remembered, Unfairly, for Banning Six Indians in South Africa, 2001–02" www.cricketcountry.com/articles/mike-denness-english-captain-remembered-unfairly-for-banning-six-indians-in-south-africa-2001-02-25437 (accessed 23rd February 2021)

178. Arunabha Sengupta, "Denness the Menace—India's Problems with Match Referee Mike Denness" http://cricmash.com/conflicts-controversies/2015/1/25/denness-the-menace-indias-problems-with-match-referee-mike-denness (accessed 23rd February 2021)
179. Kanta Murali, "The End of a Controversy" https://frontline.thehindu.com/other/article30215607.ece (accessed 23rd February 2021)
180. James Astill, *The Great Tamasha-Cricket, Corruption and the Turbulent Rise of Modern India* (Bloomsbury Publishing, 2013)
181. Ibid p. 98, See also A Cricketing View, "Bhogle, Haigh and the Great Tamasha" https://cricketingview.blogspot.com/2013/09/bhogle-haigh-and-great-tamasha.html (accessed 23rd February 2021)
182. India Today Web Desk, "India Cricketers to Be Now Tested by National Anti-Doping Agency" www.indiatoday.in/sports/cricket/story/bcci-under-ambit-of-nada-india-cricketers-to-be-tested-by-national-anti-doping-agency-1579127-2019-08-09 (accessed 23rd February 2021)
183. Akshay Ramesh, "Why the BCCI Was Reluctant to Become NADA Compliant" www.indiatoday.in/sports/cricket/story/bcci-nada-compliant-reasons-for-reluctance-india-cricket-whereabouts-quality-doping-officers-blood-tests-1579274-2019-08-09 (accessed 23rd February 2021)
184. National Anti Doping Agency, "About Us" www.nadaindia.org/en/about-us (accessed 23rd February 2021)
185. Outlook Web Bureau, "World Anti-Doping Agency Urges ICC to Resolve BCCI-NADA Stand-Off" www.outlookindia.com/website/story/wada-threatens-icc-with-anti-doping-compliance-committee-intervention-over-bcci-nada-stand-off/317414 (accessed 23rd February 2021)
186. IIPRD Blog—Intellectual Property Discussions, "BCCI Comes Under the Ambit of NADA; ICC Finally a WADA Compliant, But What Next?" https://iiprd.wordpress.com/2020/04/06/bcci-comes-under-the-ambit-of-nada-icc-finally-a-wada-compliant-but-what-next/?utm_source=Mondaq&utm_medium=syndication&utm_campaign=LinkedIn-integration (accessed 23rd February 2021)
187. Rustam Sethna, "Anti-Doping Regulation in Indian Cricket: Should the BCCI Accede to NADA's Jurisdiction?" https://sportslaw.in/home/2018/10/01/restructuring-indian-football/ (accessed 23rd February 2021)
188. PTI, "BCCI Finally Comes Under NADA, First Step Towards Becoming National Sports Federation" https://timesofindia.indiatimes.com/sports/cricket/news/bcci-finally-comes-under-nada-officially-becomes-national-sports-federation/articleshow/70602918.cms (accessed 23rd February 2021)
189. Venkata Krishna B, "BCCI Comes Under NADA Code, but Not National Sports Federation yet" www.newindianexpress.com/sport/cricket/2019/aug/10/bcci-comes-under-nada-code-but-not-national-sports-federation-yet-2016906.html (accessed 23rd February 2021)
190. "Board of Control for Cricket in India Independent Anti-Doping Tribunal Decision in the Case of Mr Pradeep Sangwan" https://icc-static-files.s3.amazonaws.com/ICC/document/2017/04/17/71eaef5d-8d0c-4367-bdde-73be74f07442/bcci-v.-sangwan-decision.pdf (accessed 24th February 2021)
191. Ibid para 4
192. World-Anti Doping Agency (n 127)
193. Board of Control for Cricket in India (n 190) para 4–5
194. Ibid para 21
195. Ibid para 61
196. Board of Control for Cricket in India (n 190) para 67
197. Ibid para 73

198. Ibid para 76
199. Ibid para 77
200. Ibid para 79
201. Ibid
202. World-Anti Doping Agency (n 127)
203. World Anti-Doping Agency (n 63) [Article 10.5.2 No Significant Fault or Negligence If an Athlete or other Person establishes in an individual case that he or she bears No Significant Fault or Negligence, then the otherwise applicable period of Ineligibility may be reduced, but the reduced period of Ineligibility may not be less than one-half of the period of Ineligibility otherwise applicable. If the otherwise applicable period of Ineligibility is a lifetime, the reduced period under this Article may be no less than eight (8) years. When a Prohibited Substance or its Markers or Metabolites is detected in an Athlete's Sample in violation of Article 2.1 (Presence of a Prohibited Substance or its Metabolites or Markers), the Athlete must also establish how the Prohibited Substance entered his or her system in order to have the period of Ineligibility reduced.]
204. CAS 2014/A/3559 para 96–99
205. Ibid
206. "Decision of Board of Control for Cricket in India Under Article 8.3 of the BCCI Anti-Doping Rules in the Case of Mr. Yusuf Pathan" http://relaunch-live.s3.amazonaws.com/cms/documents/5a545bd1e9ea8-Decision%20of%20BCCI%20in%20the%20ADRV%20Case%20of%20Mr%20Y%20Pathan.pdf (accessed 24th February 2021)
207. World Anti-Doping Agency, "Prohibited at All Times" www.wada-ama.org/en/content/what-is-prohibited/prohibited-at-all-times/beta-2-agonists (accessed 24th February 2021)
208. Decision of Board of Control for Cricket (n 206) para 3
209. Ibid para 26
210. Ibid
211. Ibid
212. Ibid
213. Ibid
214. Ibid para 28
215. CAS 2017/A/5301 and CAS 2017/A/5302
216. CAS 2017/A/5301 and CAS 2017/A/5302 (n 215) para 198
217. World-Anti Doping Agency (n 103)
218. CAS 2017/A/5301 and CAS 2017/A/5302 (n 215) 193
219. Decision of Board of Control for Cricket (n 206) para 28–29
220. "Decision of Board of Control for Cricket in India Under Article 8.3 of the BCCI Anti-Doping Rules in the Case of Mr Abhishek Gupta" https://pulse-static-files.s3.amazonaws.com/ICC/document/2018/07/05/e8f7a114-e128-4761-afe4-e9c5704eb24e/Decision-of-BCCI-in-the-ADRV-Case-of-A-Gupta.pdf (accessed 24th February 2021)
221. World Anti-Doping Agency (n 207)
222. Decision of Board of Control for Cricket (n 220) para 4
223. Decision of Board of Control for Cricket (n 206)
224. Decision of Board of Control for Cricket (n 220) para 3
225. Ibid para 14
226. Ibid
227. Ibid para 20
228. CAS 2017/A/5301 (n 215)
229. Decision of Board of Control for Cricket (n 220) para 22
230. Ibid para 22

231. Ibid
232. Ibid para 23
233. "Decision of Board of Control for Cricket in India Under Article 8.3 of the BCCI Anti-Doping Rules in the Case of Mr Akshay Dullarwar" http://relaunch-live.s3.amazonaws.com/cms/documents/5d403d05f1784-Decision%20of%20BCCI%20in%20the%20ADRV%20Case%20of%20Akshay%20Dullarwar.pdf (accessed 24th February 2021)
234. World Anti-Doping Agency, "World Anti-Doping Code International Standard Prohibited List 2021" www.wada-ama.org/sites/default/files/resources/files/2021list_en.pdf (accessed 24th February 2021)
235. Decision of Board of Control for Cricket (n 233) para 3
236. Ibid
237. Ibid para 4
238. Ibid para 20
239. Ibid
240. Ibid para 21
241. Decision of Board of Control for Cricket (n 233) para 22
242. "Decision of Board of Control for Cricket in India Under Article 8.3 of the BCCI Anti-Doping Rules in the Case of Mr Divya Gajraj" http://relaunch-live.s3.amazonaws.com/cms/documents/5d403ce913931-Decision%20of%20BCCI%20in%20the%20ADRV%20Case%20of%20Divya%20Gajraj.pdf (accessed 24th February 2021)
243. Ibid para 2
244. Ibid para 3
245. World-Anti Doping Agency (n 96)
246. Decision of Board of Control for Cricket (n 242) para 3
247. Ibid para 4
248. Ibid para 3
249. Ibid para 20
250. Ibid para 14
251. Ibid para 21
252. Ibid para 22
253. "Decision of Board of Control for Cricket in India Under Article 8.3 of the BCCI Anti-Doping Rules in the Case of Mr Prithvi Shaw" https://icc-static-files.s3.amazonaws.com/ICC/document/2019/08/04/c17bcfac-aab0-4b1c-b512-cfb3c734b103/Prithvi-Shaw.pdf (accessed 24th February 2021)
254. World Anti-Doping Agency (n 207)
255. Decision of Board of Control for Cricket (n 253) para 3
256. Ibid para 4
257. Cricbuzz, "Prithvi Shaw" cricbuzz.com/profiles/12094/prithvi-shaw#!#profile (accessed 24th February 2021)
258. Decision of Board of Control for Cricket (n 253) para 14
259. Ibid
260. Ibid para 15
261. Ibid
262. Ibid para 20
263. Decision of Board of Control for Cricket (n 253) para 21
264. Ibid para 21–22
265. Gaurav Gupta, "BCCI Runs a Robust Anti-Doping Programme: ICC" https://timesofindia.indiatimes.com/sports/cricket/news/bcci-runs-a-robust-anti-doping-programme-icc/articleshow/70529178.cms (accessed 24th February 2021)
266. World Anti-Doping Agency (n 5) [Article 12 Sanctions by Signatories Against Other Sporting Bodies Each Signatory shall adopt rules that obligate each of its

member organizations and any other sporting body over which it has authority to comply with, implement, uphold and enforce the Code within that organization's or body's area of competence. When a Signatory becomes aware that one of its member organizations or other sporting body over which it has authority has failed to fulfill such obligation, the Signatory shall take appropriate action against such organization or body.80 In particular, a Signatory's action and rules shall include the possibility of excluding all, or some group of, members of that organization or body from specified future Events or all Events conducted within a specified period of time.]

267. Ibid [Article 20.3 Roles and Responsibilities of International Federations- 20.3.2 To require, as a condition of membership, that the policies, rules and programs of their National Federations and other members are in compliance with the Code and the International Standards, and to take appropriate action to enforce such compliance; areas of compliance shall include but not be limited to: (i) requiring that their National Federations conduct Testing only under the documented authority of their International Federation and use their National Anti-Doping Organization or other Sample collection authority to collect Samples in compliance with the International Standard for Testing and Investigations; (ii) requiring that their National Federations recognize the authority of the National Anti-Doping Organization in their country in accordance with Article 5.2.1 and assist as appropriate with the National Anti-Doping Organization's implementation of the national Testing program for their sport; (iii) requiring that their National Federations analyze all Samples collected using a WADA-accredited or WADA-approved laboratory in accordance with Article 6.1; and (iv) requiring that any national level anti-doping rule violation cases discovered by their National Federations are adjudicated by an Operationally Independent hearing panel in accordance with Article 8.1 and the International Standard for Results Management.]

268. Rustam Sethna (n 187)
269. Lovely Dasgupta, *The World Anti-Doping Code-Fit for Purpose?* (Routledge, 2019)
270. National Anti-Doping Agency, "Anti-Doping Appeal Panel" www.nadaindia.org/en/antidopingappealpanel (accessed 24th February 2021)
271. PTI (n 188)
272. National Anti Doping Agency (n 184)

References

- PTI, "IOC Recognizes ICC, Cricket Can Now Become Olympic Sport" www.live mint.com/Consumer/C6ANnHs0Zbme94bLoZOf5O/IOC-recognizes-ICC-cricket-can-now-become-Olympic-sport.html (accessed 20th February 2021)
- ARISF, "Members" www.arisf.sport/members.aspx (accessed 20th February 2021)
- ICC Anti-Doping, "ICC Anti-Doping Code" www.icc-cricket.com/about/integrity/anti-doping/code (accessed 20th February 2021)
- World Anti-Doping Agency, "World Anti-Doping Code 2021" www.wada-ama.org/sites/default/files/resources/files/2021_wada_code.pdf (accessed 21 February 2021)
- International Cricket Council, "Player's Consent and Agreement to the Anti-Doping Code" https://icc-static-files.s3.amazonaws.com/ICC/document/2019/05/02/de344f3b-1ba1-4a67-b5a8-745172f7e826/ICC-Player-s-Consent-and-Agreement-form.pdf (accessed 20th February 2021)
- "National Cricket Federations Anti-Doping Rules Template Effective, 1st January 2021" https://resources.pulse.icc-cricket.com/ICC/document/2021/01/14/

c52a3589-f99d-4d5b-a078-ec97f90ce1fe/National-Cricket-Federations-Anti-Doping-Rules-Template-effective-1Jan21.pdf (accessed 20th February 2021)

- International Cricket Council (n 3) "Where Abouts Requirements for Out-of Competition Testing- Effective Date: 1 January 2021" https://resources.pulse.icc-cricket.com/ICC/document/2020/12/31/de7262c0-b6d9-4550-a2a6-ca85700292e2/Whereabouts-Regulations-effective-1-Jan-2021.pdf (accessed 20th February 2021)
- World Anti-Doping Agency, "The World Anti-Doping Code International Standard Testing and Investigations" www.wada-ama.org/sites/default/files/resources/files/international_standard_isti_-_2020.pdf (accessed 20th February 2021)
- International Cricket Council, "About Our Members" [Full Members Are the Governing Bodies for Cricket of a Country Recognised by the ICC, or Nations Associated for Cricket Purposes, or a Geographical Area, from Which Representative Teams Are Qualified to Play official Test Matches (12 Members)" www.icc-cricket.com/about/members/about-our-members (accessed 20th February 2021)
- www.wada-ama.org/en/what-we-do/international-standards (accessed 21st February 2021)
- World Anti-Doping Agency, "Athletes' Anti-Doping Rights Act [Approved by WADA's Executive Committee on 7 November 2019]" www.wada-ama.org/sites/default/files/resources/files/athlete_act_en.pdf (accessed 21st February 2021)
- ICC Anti-Doping, "Decisions and Periods of Ineligibility" www.icc-cricket.com/about/integrity/anti-doping/decisions-and-integrity (accessed 21st February 2021)
- Chinmay Jawalekar, "Upul Tharanga: 11 Facts About the Consistently Inconsistent Sri Lankan Batsman" www.cricketcountry.com/articles/upul-tharanga-11-facts-about-the-consistently-inconsistent-sri-lankan-batsman-512257 (accessed 21st February 2021)
- Cricbuzz, "Upul Tharanga Sri Lanka" www.cricbuzz.com/profiles/414/upul-tharanga#!#profile (accessed 21st February 2021)
- "International Cricket Council Independent Anti-Doping Tribunal Decision in the Case of Mr Upul Tharanga, Para 3" https://fdocuments.in/reader/full/international-cricket-council-independent-anti-doping (accessed 21st February 2021)
- World-Anti Doping Agency, "What Is Prohibited-Prohibited In-Competition" www.wada-ama.org/en/content/what-is-prohibited/prohibited-in-competition/glucocorticoids (accessed 21st February 2021)
- www.wada-ama.org/sites/default/files/resources/files/wada_anti-doping_code_2009_en_0.pdf (accessed 21st February 2021)
- CAS 2011/A/2515
- ESPNcricinfo Staff, "Treymane Smartt Suspended for Anti-Doping Violation" www.espncricinfo.com/story/west-indies-news-treymane-smartt-suspended-for-anti-doping-violation-541123 (accessed 21st February 2021)
- World-Anti Doping Agency, "Prohibited at All Times- Diuretics and Masking Agents" www.wada-ama.org/en/content/what-is-prohibited/prohibited-at-all-times/diuretics-and-masking-agents (accessed 21st February 2021)
- "International Cricket Council and Yasir Shah Disciplinary Proceedings Under the ICC Anti-Doping Code 2015" http://icc-live.s3.amazonaws.com/cms/media/about_docs/56c837d5b5413-Yasir%20Shah%20-%20Agreed%20Decision%20FINAL%2007%20February%202016%20WEBSITE.PDF (accessed 21st February 2021)

- "Significant Changes Between the 2009 Code and the 2015 Code, Version 4.0" www. wada-ama.org/sites/default/files/wadc-2015-draft-version-4.0-significant-changes-to-2009-en.pdf (accessed 22nd February 2021)
- www.wada-ama.org/sites/default/files/resources/files/wada-2015-world-anti-doping-code.pdf (accessed 22nd February 2021)
- World-Anti Doping Agency, "Prohibited List Q&A" www.wada-ama.org/en/questions-answers/prohibited-list-qa (accessed 22nd February 2021)
- "In the Matter of Proceedings Brought Under the BCB Anti-Doping Rules Between: The Bangladesh Cricket Board and Mr Kaz! Anik Islam" https://resources.pulse.icc-cricket.com/ICC/document/2020/07/27/764211fb-135d-4089-aa55-debdd1080eb3/Kazi-Anik-AD-decision.pdf (accessed 22nd February 2021)
- World-Anti Doping Agency, "World Anti-Doping Code International Standard Prohibited List" www.wada-ama.org/sites/default/files/resources/files/2021list_en.pdf (accessed 22nd February 2021)
- "Before the Sports Tribunal of New Zealand-Drug Free Sport New Zealand and Harrisyn Jones and New Zealand Cricket" https://icc-static-files.s3.amazonaws.com/ICC/document/2018/09/20/b3f51e27-455a-40d0-824c-7cdebc2b23b7/ST0518-Decision.pdf (accessed 22nd February 2021)
- "The Anti-Doping Tribunal-in the Adjudication Proceeding Between Pakistan Cricket Board (PCB) and Kashif Saddique" http://icc-live.s3.amazonaws.com/cms/media/about_docs/537498900afda-PCB%20-%20Kashif%20Siddique%20-%20 Apr%202014.pdf (accessed 22nd February 2021)
- World-Anti Doping Agency, "Prohibited at All Times" www.wada-ama.org/en/content/what-is-prohibited/prohibited-at-all-times/anabolic-agents (accessed 22nd February 2021)
- "In the Matter of Raza Hasan, Cricketer" http://icc-live.s3.amazonaws.com/cms/media/about_docs/556ab7b724b5d-In%20the%20Matter%20of%20Raza%20 Hasan%20(Cricketer).pdf (accessed 22nd February 2021)
- World-Anti Doping Agency, "Substances of Abuse Under the 2021 World Anti-Doping Code Guidance Note for Anti-Doping Organizations" www.wada-ama.org/sites/default/files/resources/files/2020-01-11_guidance_note_on_substances_of_abuse_en_0.pdf (accessed 22nd February 2021)
- The World Anti-Doping Code, "The 2015 Prohibited List International Standard" www.wada-ama.org/sites/default/files/resources/files/wada-2015-prohibited-list-en. pdf (accessed 22nd February 2021)
- ESPNcricinfo Staff, "Rehman Banned for 12 Weeks for Cannabis Use" www.espncricinfo.com/story/abdur-rehman-banned-for-12-weeks-for-cannabis-585337 (accessed 22nd February 2021)
- The World Anti-Doping Code, "The 2012 Prohibited List International Standard" www.wada-ama.org/sites/default/files/resources/files/WADA_Prohibited_List_2012_EN.pdf (accessed 22nd February 2021)
- "SA Institute For Drug Free Sport (SAIDS) Anti Doping Disciplinary Hearing: Mr Rory Kleinveldt and Cricket South Africa ('CSA')" www.doping.nl/media/kb/1439/SAIDS%20Kleinveldt%202012-07%20(S).pdf (accessed 22nd February 2021)
- "The Jamaica Anti-Doping Disciplinary Panel Between Jamaica Anti-Doping Commission and Odean Brown" http://icc-live.s3.amazonaws.com/cms/media/about_docs/578612fba01e6-OdeanBrown.pdf (accessed 22nd February 2021)

- BCCI, "About the BCCI" www.bcci.tv/about/history (accessed 23rd February 2021)
- Sportskeeda, "For Cricket to Grow Globally, BCCI's Power Needs to Be Curtailed: Part 1" https://cricket.yahoo.net/news/for-cricket-grow-globally-bcci-s-power-needs-curtailed-part-1 (accessed 23rd February 2021)
- Shamik Chakrabarty, "India Is a Global Power in Cricket . . . Position Cannot Be Compromised: BCCI Secretary Ajay Shirke" https://indianexpress.com/article/sports/cricket/india-global-power-cricket-position-cannot-compromised-bcci-secretary-ajay-shirke-3023340/ (accessed 23rd February 2021)
- Aswathi R. Jayachandran, "BCCI-ICC: The Tug of Financial War" https://medium.com/crimpulse/bcci-icc-the-tug-of-financial-war-fddf2a540696 (accessed 23rd February 2021)
- Team Bridge, "In India Cricket Is a Religion, as Football Is in European Countries" https://thebridge.in/latest/india-cricket-religion-football-in-european-countries/#:~:text=Mecca%20of%20making%20money!&text=Thus%2C%20cricket%20is%20not%20only,has%20generated%20loads%20of%20revenue (accessed 23rd February 2021)
- Worldometer, "India Population" www.worldometers.info/world-population/india-population/ (accessed 23rd February 2021)
- Martin Williamson, "How the World Cup Became a Commercial Hit" www.espncricinfo.com/story/martin-williamson-how-the-world-cup-became-a-commercial-hit-824079 (accessed 23rd February 2021)
- https://twitter.com/mohanstatsman/status/981897579226165248 (accessed 23rd February 2021)
- Ashish Magotra, "From 1983's Miracle Win to Financial Might of IPL: How India Increased Control Over World Cricket" https://scroll.in/field/958713/from-1983s-miracle-win-to-financial-might-of-ipl-how-india-increased-control-over-world-cricket (accessed 23rd February 2021)
- Venkat Ananth, "How BCCI Became the 800-Pound Gorilla of Cricket" www.livemint.com/Consumer/pVdCJRSBBid7eVxuCwfqcK/How-India-became-the-800-pound-gorilla-of-cricket.html (accessed 23rd February 2021)
- Sharda Ugra, "Match Referee Mike Denness' Harsh Sentences Pitch BCCI into Confrontation with ICC" www.indiatoday.in/magazine/cover-story/story/20011203-match-referee-mike-denness-harsh-sentences-pitch-bcci-into-confrontation-with-icc-774971-2001-12-03 (accessed 23rd February 2021)
- Martin Williamson, "The Denness Affair" www.espncricinfo.com/magazine/content/story/496743.html (accessed 23rd February 2021)
- V.S. Aravind, "Denness the Menace- When Tendulkar Was Called 'Cheat'" www.sify.com/sports/denness-the-menace-when-tendulkar-was-called-cheat-news-cricket-pj2qbrhddgjfb.html (accessed 23rd February 2021)
- Aabhas Sharma, "Jagmohan Dalmiya: The Man Who Showed Who Is the Boss" www.rediff.com/cricket/report/jagmohan-dalmiya-the-man-who-showed-who-is-the-boss-bcci-sachin-tendulkar-ball-tampering-pix/20150922.htm (accessed 23rd February 2021)
- Arunabha Sengupta, "Mike Denness: English Captain Remembered, Unfairly, for Banning Six Indians in South Africa, 2001–02" www.cricketcountry.com/articles/mike-denness-english-captain-remembered-unfairly-for-banning-six-indians-in-south-africa-2001-02-25437 (accessed 23rd February 2021)
- Arunabha Sengupta, "Denness the Menace—India's Problems with Match Referee Mike Denness" http://cricmash.com/conflicts-controversies/2015/1/25/

denness-the-menace-indias-problems-with-match-referee-mike-denness (accessed 23rd February 2021)

- Kanta Murali, "The End of a Controversy" https://frontline.thehindu.com/other/article30215607.ece (accessed 23rd February 2021)
- James Astill, *The Great Tamasha-Cricket, Corruption and the Turbulent Rise of Modern India* (Bloomsbury Publishing, 2013)
- A Cricketing View, "Bhogle, Haigh and the Great Tamasha" https://cricketing-view.blogspot.com/2013/09/bhogle-haigh-and-great-tamasha.html (accessed 23rd February 2021)
- India Today Web Desk, "India Cricketers to Be Now Tested by National Anti-Doping Agency" www.indiatoday.in/sports/cricket/story/bcci-under-ambit-of-nada-india-cricketers-to-be-tested-by-national-anti-doping-agency-1579127-2019-08-09 (accessed 23rd February 2021)
- Akshay Ramesh, "Why the BCCI Was Reluctant to Become NADA Compliant" www.indiatoday.in/sports/cricket/story/bcci-nada-compliant-reasons-for-reluctance-india-cricket-whereabouts-quality-doping-officers-blood-tests-1579274-2019-08-09 (accessed 23rd February 2021)
- National Anti Doping Agency, "About Us" www.nadaindia.org/en/about-us (accessed 23rd February 2021)
- Outlook Web Bureau, "World Anti-Doping Agency Urges ICC to Resolve BCCI-NADA Stand-Off" www.outlookindia.com/website/story/wada-threatens-icc-with-anti-doping-compliance-committee-intervention-over-bcci-nada-stand-off/317414 (accessed 23rd February 2021)
- IIPRD Blog—Intellectual Property Discussions, "BCCI Comes Under the Ambit of NADA; ICC Finally a Wada Compliant, but What Next?" https://iiprd.wordpress.com/2020/04/06/bcci-comes-under-the-ambit-of-nada-icc-finally-a-wada-compliant-but-what-next/?utm_source=Mondaq&utm_medium=syndication&utm_campaign=LinkedIn-integration (accessed 23rd February 2021)
- Rustam Sethna, "Anti-Doping Regulation in Indian Cricket: Should the BCCI Accede to NADA's Jurisdiction?" https://sportslaw.in/home/2018/10/01/restructuring-indian-football/ (accessed 23rd February 2021)
- PTI, "BCCI Finally Comes Under NADA, First Step Towards Becoming National Sports Federation" https://timesofindia.indiatimes.com/sports/cricket/news/bcci-finally-comes-under-nada-officially-becomes-national-sports-federation/articleshow/70602918.cms (accessed 23rd February 2021)
- Venkata Krishna B, "BCCI Comes Under NADA Code, but not National Sports Federation yet" www.newindianexpress.com/sport/cricket/2019/aug/10/bcci-comes-under-nada-code-but-not-national-sports-federation-yet-2016906.html (accessed 23rd February 2021)
- "Board of Control for Cricket in India Independent Anti-Doping Tribunal Decision in the Case of Mr Pradeep Sangwan" https://icc-static-files.s3.amazonaws.com/ICC/document/2017/04/17/71eaef5d-8d0c-4367-bdde-73be74f07442/bcci-v.-sangwan-decision.pdf (accessed 24th February 2021)
- CAS 2014/A/3559
- "Decision of Board of Control for Cricket in India Under Article 8.3 of the BCCI Anti-Doping Rules in the Case of Mr. Yusuf Pathan" http://relaunch-live.s3.amazonaws.com/cms/documents/5a545bd1e9ea8-Decision%20of%20BCCI%20in%20the%20ADRV%20Case%20of%20Mr%20Y%20Pathan.pdf (accessed 24th February 2021)

- World Anti-Doping Agency, "Prohibited at All Times" www.wada-ama.org/en/content/what-is-prohibited/prohibited-at-all-times/beta-2-agonists (accessed 24th February 2021)
- CAS 2017/A/530 & CAS 2017/A/5302
- "Decision of Board of Control for Cricket in India Under Article 8.3 of the BCCI Anti-Doping Rules in the Case of Mr Abhishek Gupta" https://pulse-static-files.s3.amazonaws.com/ICC/document/2018/07/05/e8f7a114-e128-4761-afe4-e9c5704eb24e/Decision-of-BCCI-in-the-ADRV-Case-of-A-Gupta.pdf (accessed 24th February 2021)
- "Decision of Board of Control for Cricket in India Under Article 8.3 of the BCCI Anti-Doping Rules in the Case of Mr Akshay Dullarwar" http://relaunch-live.s3.amazonaws.com/cms/documents/5d403d05f1784-Decision%20of%20BCCI%20in%20the%20ADRV%20Case%20of%20Akshay%20Dullarwar.pdf (accessed 24th February 2021)
- World Anti-Doping Agency, "World Anti-Doping Code International Standard Prohibited List 2021" www.wada-ama.org/sites/default/files/resources/files/2021list_en.pdf (accessed 24th February 2021)
- "Decision of Board of Control for Cricket in India Under Article 8.3 of the BCCI Anti-Doping Rules in the Case of Mr Divya Gajraj" http://relaunch-live.s3.amazonaws.com/cms/documents/5d403ce913931-Decision%20of%20BCCI%20in%20the%20ADRV%20Case%20of%20Divya%20Gajraj.pdf (accessed 24th February 2021)
- "Decision of Board of Control for Cricket in India Under Article 8.3 of the BCCI Anti-Doping Rules in the Case of Mr Prithvi Shaw" https://icc-static-files.s3.amazonaws.com/ICC/document/2019/08/04/c17bcfac-aab0-4b1c-b512-cfb3c734b103/Prithvi-Shaw.pdf (accessed 24th February 2021)
- Cricbuzz, "Prithvi Shaw" cricbuzz.com/profiles/12094/prithvi-shaw#!#profile (accessed 24th February 2021)
- Gaurav Gupta, "BCCI Runs a Robust Anti-Doping Programme: ICC" https://timesofindia.indiatimes.com/sports/cricket/news/bcci-runs-a-robust-anti-doping-programme-icc/articleshow/70529178.cms (accessed 24th February 2021)
- Lovely Dasgupta, *The World Anti-Doping Code-Fit for Purpose?* (Routledge, 2019)
- National Anti-Doping Agency, "Anti-Doping Appeal Panel" www.nadaindia.org/en/antidopingappealpanel (accessed 24th February 2021)

5 Relationship of Dance Sport and Anti-Doping

Introduction

Dance sport does not invoke the images of doping; however, it does have a serious problem in this area. There are empirical research works done, which highlight the prevalence of substance abuse and doping in Dance sport. This chapter takes up the sport primarily because of its uniqueness. For not many would consider Dance as a sport. Further, Dance sport is different from other sports primarily because it is a generic term that includes different forms of dance within its ambit. Lastly, Dance sport has been in the public sphere for long and accordingly has also got the attention of the International Olympic Committee (IOC). Accordingly, Dance sport is one of the oldest recognized Non-Olympic sport. Despite the length for which Dance sport has enjoyed the status of a Non-Olympic sport, it has yet to join the Olympic program. Another factor that needs to be analyzed is the process of recognition of Dance sport as a Non-Olympic sport. This is so because of the relatively easier terms and conditions that prevailed at the time when Dance sport was recognized by IOC. At the time when Dance sport got recognition, there was no compulsion to have a robust anti-doping program in place. Accordingly, the parameters of recognition were not focused on this aspect of the governance of the sport. Dance sport, comparatively had it easy in terms of getting recognized as a Non-Olympic sport. Another interesting bit about Dance sport is the multiplicity of Governing Bodies (GB) that were initially in charge of the sport. The body recognized by the IOC is different from the current organization in charge of Dance sport. And that calls for an interesting study into Dance sport as a Non-Olympic sport. Considering that it continues to campaign for inclusion in the Olympic program, the claim needs to be tested. The chapter begins by analyzing the evolution of Dance from Art to sport. The process through which the sport went on to achieve its current form as a Non-Olympic sport. The governance issues led to the multiple changes of the guard in terms of the official International Federation (IF) in charge. The next section of the chapter looks at the prevalence of doping within dance sport. The IF currently in charge of the sport enforces the anti-doping program. The rules and regulations were used to enforce the anti-doping program. Then, it looks into the impact of the adoption

DOI: 10.4324/9781003082309-5

of the World Anti-Doping Agency (WADA) Code on the Dance sport. The analyses involve the study of the impact that compliance requirement within the WADA Code is likely to have on a relatively small International Federation. Importantly, the WADA Code compliance issue with the Dance sport is also looked into because of its largely Euro-centric origin. The chapter then looks into the extent to which the concerned IF has been lax in implementing the WADA Code. The matter is analyzed on the basis of the empirical report generated on this issue by various researchers. The same is also done through the few cases that have been discussed and debated before CAS. The chapter argues that the implementation of the WADA Code within a small federation is a feasible proposition if the members are not struggling for funds and there are no other structural constraints. Importantly, the recognition process of smaller IFs should ensure that there is effective compliance with the WADA Code. Being a relatively older Non-Olympic sport, Dance sport should develop a robust compliance mechanism. Both World Anti-Doping Agency (WADA) and IOC should test the compliance level when they review the recognition granted to such sports. Importantly, such testing needs to be done more stringently when the sport is proposed to be included in the Olympic program.

From Dance to Sport—Teething Issues With Governance

The transition from Dance to sport is to be credited to the Europeans. The rules, regulations, and norms that would sustain the activity as sports were accordingly laid down. A concerted effort was made to have an integrated governance structure for the activity to be promoted as a Dance sport. In 1929, the Britishers established a style called the "English style" and laid down the standard for the same. It was this style of Dance that gained popularity elsewhere. The formalization of a governing body to administer and regulate the Dance sport was done by the Germans. The German Imperial Association for the Fostering of Social Dance was responsible for establishing the Fédération Internationale de Danse pour Amateurs (FIDA).[1] FIDA had nine founding members, all from Europe. They established FIDA on 10th September 1935 in Prague. The first world championship, under the aegis of FIDA, was conducted a year later in Bad Nauheim, Germany.[2] FIDA was, however, plagued with the problem of conflicts between amateur and professional dancers. Accordingly, it could survive only for 20 years, suspending all its activities in 1956. Germans were once more at the forefront of the activities leading to the formation of a new organization. Hence on 12th May, at the residence of German Dance Champion Otto Teipel, eight European nations started the International Council of Amateur Dancers (ICAD). Teipel became the first president of the ICAD, which expanded a year later to include four more nations under its wing. However, as in the case of FIDA, ICAD too faced difficulties in its attempt to reconcile with the organization of Professional Dance.[3]

The problems plaguing FIDA thus did not disappear in the case of ICAD and that took a toll on Teipel. He stepped down as President of ICAD worn out by the continuous strife and dispute between amateur and professional danc-ers. He was succeeded by Heinrich Brönner and Rolf Fincke, both having a short-lived tenure. It was under the leadership of Detlef Hegemann the tus-sle between amateur and professional dancers got resolved. Under his leader-ship, ICAD signed a historical agreement with the International Council of Ballroom Dancing (ICBD). The agreement called the "Bremen Agreement" signed on October 3, 1965, clearly demarcated the operational area of ICAD and ICBD.[4] It was thus decided that ICAD will regulate and conduct interna-tional championships for the amateurs and ICBD will conduct similar events for the professionals. Post this agreement, ICAD successfully expanded its membership base. Several nations across the world joined in to promote and practice amateur Dance sport. ICAD promoted the sport for 25 years nurturing its growth. In 1990, to ensure wider acceptance of the Dance sport, ICAD was rechristened as International Dance Sport Federation (IDSF). The change in the name made the sport more familiar to the consuming public. Consequently, the IDSF attracted larger membership as well as patronage for the sports.[5]

The name firmly established the idea of Dance as a sport irrespective of its form or style. As the sport grew, its acceptability as well as popularity grew. In 1992, IDSF was granted the membership of the Global Association of Interna-tional Sports Federation (GAISF).[6] GAISF is an umbrella organization for all the International Sports Federations (IFs). It extends membership to all IFs irre-spective of their status as recognized or un-recognized sports. Hence, IDSF's inclusion in GAISF legitimized their claim as a sport that had the potential of becoming a recognized sport.[7] It was a seal of approval for the norms that had been laid down to structure the activity as sport. IDSF thus became a legitimate IF. And this legitimacy emboldened IDSF to apply for the recognition by Inter-national Olympic Committee (IOC). They were successful in gaining provi-sional recognition from the IOC in 1995. In the same year, the IDSF joined the International World Games Association (IWGA).[8] The purpose of the IWGA is to organize multidisciplinary events covering the sports of all its members. The IWGA thus aims to promote and popularize the sports of its members.[9] The IDSF thus achieved an important milestone by getting admitted to IWGA. In 1997, the IDSF achieved the important milestone of getting full recognition from the IOC and also got the membership of the Association of IOC Recog-nized International Sports Federations (ARISF).[10] Thus, IDSF's journey as a legitimate IF and Dance sport as a legitimate sport culminated successfully. Though the governance issues were there in the initial stage, the same has got firmly resolved with the formal recognition of IOC. It is the only recognized IF for all forms of Dance sport. Hence, gradually all the other organizations dealing with Dance merged with IDSF. IDSF's dominance and control over the sport are evident from the fact that in 2007 it was instrumental in the formation of the International Professional Dance Sport Council (IPDSC).[11]

IPDSC had a close collaboration with the IDSF in all matters relating to the governance of the sport. In 2010, however, IPDSC got dissolved and merged with the IDSF. Consequently, IDSF created a professional Dance sport division responsible for organizing tournaments for the professionals. In 2011, IDSF was re-christened as World Dance Sport Federation (WDSF). WDSF is thus presently the official IF for Dance sport (both amateurs and professionals).[12] The WDSF is responsible for the promotion and organization of tournaments for Dance sport. WDSF is also responsible for the due discharge of all its responsibilities as undertaken toward the IOC. Accordingly, it is responsible for fulfilling its compliance obligations. WDSF is responsible to ensure that its members also fulfill the commitment undertaken at the time of grant of recognition. WDSF is thus responsible for ensuring the effective implementation of the anti-doping regulations. WDSF, like its predecessor, has to increase the following of the Dance sport. Considering that Dance sport dreams of being included in the Olympic Games, WDSF has an important task of ensuring effective WADA Code compliance. WDSF has to build up on the popularity that exists vis-à-vis the sport among its members. As per the WDSF website, currently there are 91 countries that are members of the WDSF.[13] And the membership crisscrosses across the Continents and not confined only to the European countries. This establishes the growing popularity of the sport and thus it becomes essential to assess its anti-doping compliance. It also becomes necessary to understand the attitude of WDSF towards anti-doping regulations.

Anti-Doping Compliance, WDSF, and IOC: Testing the Recognition Process

The WDSF (formerly the IDSF) was granted provisional recognition by the IOC in the year 1995.[14] The IOC Charter of 1995 did not have much in terms of the requirements that an IF needed to fulfill to be recognized.[15] As per Rule 29 of the IOC Charter, the recognition of an IF, not part of the Olympic movement, was at the whims and fancies of the IOC.[16] For the IOC did not lay down any criteria to be looked into for the grant of such recognition. Further, the recognition was provisional and was to lapse at the end of 2 years. It could go beyond 2 years if the original grant of recognition had mentioned a period greater than 2 years. The provisional recognition could be full and permanent if the IOC confirmed the same in writing.[17] On the whole, what mattered was lobbying with the IOC and not any other criteria pertaining to compliance. This makes life easy for the IFs seeking recognition of the IOC. Further, the narrative becomes even more ambiguous as we come across Rule 52. It states emphatically that only Olympic sports can be part of the Olympic Games.[18] In such a scenario, the IFs getting recognized under Rule 29 has no scope of becoming an Olympic sport if the recognition lapses at the end of 2 years. Apart from these two Rules, the 1995 Charter has no other Rules having a bearing on the recognition of an IF. Against this background, it is evident that the recognition of the IDSF (now WDSF) was not based on any stringent criteria. Evidently, it was lobbying that convinced the IOC to grant it a provisional recognition for 2 years.

A perusal of the minutes of the 106th Session of the IOC held at Lausanne, from September 2 to 6, 1997, details the reasons for recognizing IDSF (herein-after called WDSF).[19] As per the minutes of the said meeting, full recognition for WDSF was recommended without any discussion as to the reasons for the same.[20] Interestingly, the said minutes of the session also reveals the sad state of affairs with respect to the compliance with the Charter, within Olympic sports. As noted therein many of the National Olympic Committees (NOC) failed to comply with the essentials of the Olympic Charter.[21] At the relevant time, the only essential mandates of the Olympic Charter were the Olympic Medical Code and the Court of Arbitration for Sport (CAS).[22] Hence, one can understand that the pressure on a Non-Olympic sport was negligible. Thus, WDSF had a cakewalk in terms of compliance with the Olympic Charter. More so because the world of sports was yet to experience a major shakeup as a result of lax anti-doping compliances. Therefore, it is not surprising that the shock came from within the Olympic sports. On July 8, 1998, the world of sports was rocked by the Festina affair.[23] It involved trafficking, possession, and use of performance-enhancing drugs.[24] The entire narrative of the anti-doping regulation changed. IOC was left fumbling for answers. And the exist-ing anti-doping program run by the IOC Medical Commission was exposed. This was the major event that forced the world of sports to re-think its method of enforcing anti-doping regulations. That was the trigger that led to the estab-lishment of the World Anti-Doping Agency (WADA). And since then the IOC mandates compliance with WADA as a pre-requisite for getting recognized.[25]

This background is important for it highlights the fact that WDSF has had it easy when it comes to recognition by the IOC. The lack of stringency has had an impact on the compliance level of WDSF. As of date, there are very few reported cases of ADRV within sports. As will be seen later, the lesser number of reported cases does not lead to a conclusion that the sports are clean. The WDSF also fails on account of transparency for the website is largely about the achievements of the sports persons. It does not give any information about compliance with the WADA Code or the outcome. The WDSF website has information on its rules and regulations as well as the competitions but noth-ing on the extent to which the athletes or the members are in compliance. The information is basic and the only substantial thing is that it gets updated with the revision of the WADA Code. Thus, the current WDSF regulations are in accordance with the WADA Code 2021.[26] However, such compliance on paper does not mean anything in real terms. Neither does it prove that WDSF is strin-gently compliant with the WADA Code. It does not create any presumption in favor of the athletes either that they refrain from the use of the prohibited substances. Similarly, it does not create a presumption in favor of the members that they too are in compliance with the WADA Code. The WDSF website does have a section that has information on the sample tested. However, the data uploaded in this section were last updated in the year 2017. Hence, that too reflects poorly on the WDSF's compliance record. A study of the WDSF's

Anti-Doping regulation as well as its implementation might provide some clue toward its compliance efforts.

Anti-Doping Code and WDSF-Knotty Affair

The WDSF (formerly IDSF) has, on paper, incorporated the WADA Code in their own Anti-Doping Code.[27] As specified in the WADA Code, herein too the WDSF in charge of conducting all aspects of doping control.[28] The WDSF Code is meant to apply to all the members and athletes of WDSF.[29] As per Article 5 of the WDSF STATUTES, it is mandatory for the members to agree to comply with both the WADA Code and the WDSF Anti-Doping Code.[30] Further Article 21 declares that the Anti-Doping Code is an integral part of the WDSF STATUTES.[31] The Anti-Doping Code has, in keeping with the standard prescribed by the WADA Code, adopted the principle of strict liability,[32] subject to the mitigating factors. Further, the standard and burden of proof remain that of balance of probability for the athletes and comfortable satisfaction of the Panel for the IF, viz., WDSF.[33] Similarly, the WDSF has adopted the prohibited list as published under the WADA Code.[34] The other rules pertaining to Therapeutic Use Exemption (TUE), whereabouts filing, sample testing, and result management are taken as it is from WADA Code.[35] In addition, the procedure for conducting hearing, sanction, and appeal to CAS is also provided for and is the same as that in WADA Code.[36] The professional division of the WDSF is also governed by this Code. The rules and regulations as available on the WDSF website for the professional division do not provide for separate Anti-Doping Code. Hence, it has to be assumed that Anti-Doping regulations are common to both amateur and professional dancers. Understandably so since the WADA Code itself does not make any distinction between amateur and professionals.[37]

As mentioned earlier, in almost 24 years of its existence, WDSF has till date reported very few cases of ADRV. The WDSF has established a Disciplinary Council, which is an autonomous adjudicatory body. It has been conferred with the power to adjudicate upon, among others, matters arising from the breach of the WDSF Anti-Doping Code.[38] And the Council has till date, as per the WDSF website, adjudicated eight cases. The first case involved Edita Daniute,[39] who was sanctioned for a period of 3 months. The decision was rendered in the year 2006 for the ADRV caused by the presence of Sibutramine, a stimulant. The Council went into the discussion on the degree of fault of the athlete who pleaded in-advertent doping. The Council looked into the publicly available information. And the Council pointed out that a simple internet search would have revealed the composition of the medication that the athlete used. Commenting on the degree of fault of the athlete the Council commented that

> the Athlete cannot claim ignorance as . . . the information on the substance, effects of the substance, on the combination specifically with Meizitang are easily accessible to any person and of course much more accessible to

an Athlete who should be informed about the drugs and other substances she takes.[40]

However, the Council, based on scientific evidence, found that the substance consumed by the athlete had more negative effects than positive. The negative effects were significant enough to rule out any performance-enhancing benefits to the athlete.[41] Further, the Council did not rule out the possibility of inadvertent doping. In totality of the circumstances, the sanction period was reduced to 3 months.[42]

In the case of Ivan Novikov, the Council gave a decision of not guilty in favor of the athlete. The argument of the governing body that the athlete evaded doping control test could not be established. The fault was of the WDSF to not provide notice of doping control test in a language that the athlete can understand. The notice was in German, whereas it ought to have been in English. Since the official language of the WDSF is English. Further, there was no proper supervision over the athlete and there were no further instructions given to the athlete for providing an additional sample. In totality of the circumstances, no ADRV was established here.[43] In the case of Boris Maltsev and Zarina Shamsutdinova, the Council held the athletes to be guilty of ADRV for having refused to submit to the Doping control test.[44] The sanction period was reduced to one year on the ground of No Significant Fault or Negligence. Primarily because the Council found that there were lapses on the part of the organizing committee of the event where the test was conducted.[45] In the case of Olga Shcherbina, the Council imposed an ineligibility period of one year on the ground of No Significant Fault or Negligence.[46] The ADRV was caused due to the presence of acetazolamide, a diuretic, listed on the Prohibited List of the WADA Code.[47] Being a case of ingestion of a specified substance, the Council looked into the degree of fault and intention to cheat. The Council did not consider the conduct of the Athlete as reasonable or diligent.[48] However, weighing in the fact that the negative effects were greater than any performance-enhancing effect, the period of ineligibility was reduced.[49]

In the case of Flora Bouchereau,[50] the ADRV was caused by the presence of Morphine, a specified substance and banned in-competition.[51] The athlete pleaded inadvertent doping without the intention to cheat. The source was claimed to be the medicine that the athlete was taking.[52] The Council held it to be a case of No Significant Fault or Negligence and accordingly reduced the sanction to a period of one year. The Council noted that

> the Athlete . . . just did not think of committing a violation of an anti-doping rule by taking the medication, it still must be considered at least as significant negligence that the Athlete did not remember consulting the Prohibited List and asking for a TUE in the present case.[53]

The sanction was backdated keeping in mind the delay and laches on the part of the WDSF. The outcome was that the athlete was to effectively serve an ineligibility period of one month.[54] In the case of Elizaveta Yuryevna Cherev-ichnaya,[55] ADRV was caused due to the presence of furosemide, a diuretics, and masking agents, and is banned at all times by WADA.[56] However, it is a specified substance and as per the Council "the Athlete explained how this substance entered her body, the Chamber in Charge may assess if the conditions for a reduction of the period of ineligibility are given."[57] And the Council upon analyses of the facts as well as the jurisprudence on the issue held that the athlete is an

> experienced dancer . . . their knowledge of such important documents as the World Anti-Doping Code and the Prohibited List must be expected . . . she took furosemide the day before the competition . . . which creates a purposeful nexus between the ingestion of furosemide and the Athlete's competition . . . the Athlete's conduct must be assessed as gross negligence.[58]

The outcome of this analysis was that the Council did not reduce the penalty but imposed an ineligibility period of 2 years.[59]

The last case reported on the WDSF website on ADRV is Vitaly Panteleev and Angelina Nechkhaeva.[60] In this case, the ADRV was due to the presence of "Heptaminol and 1,3-dimethylbutylamine (DMBA), both banned stimulants, under Section 6 of the World Anti-Doping Agency 2017 Prohibited List, such list having been adopted by the World Dance Sport Federation in 2016."[61] The athlete failed to prove how the substance entered their system. Hence, there was the possibility of the athlete deliberately taking the prohibited substance to increase performance.[62] Accordingly, no mitigating ground could be applied herein. The period of ineligibility imposed was 2 years,[63] as applicable for ingestion of specified substances under the WADA Code 2015.[64] Thus, the WDSF has applied the WADA Code over the years through the few cases on ADRV. However, one needs to note that of the eight cases, most of them were met with the reduced penalty. Further, in many of the cases, the athlete pleaded inadvertent doping and the same was accepted. Finally, the Council did read through the CAS jurisprudence to substantiate its reasoning. This indicates that the Council is ready to apply stringent rules for ADRV; however, it still gives the benefit of doubt to the athlete wherever possible. The cases also reveal that WDSF and its members are not always prompt in their response toward a case of ADRV. There have been delays and laches on the part of the WDSF and that in turn benefits the athlete. Especially, where the penalty is reduced and then is backdated taking into account the lapses on the part of the WDSF. However, as mentioned earlier, the WDSF has not been able to successfully handle the menace of ADRV as will be seen next.

Doping the Dance and WDSF-Messing With WADA Code

Dance by becoming a sport transcended the boundaries of art and became treated as a regulated and organized activity.[65] In doing so, Dance sport blurred the line between art and sport, especially competitive sport.[66] Since modern sport is about competition, Dance sport inevitably fell into the trappings of competition.[67] The Dance sport has nonetheless maintained a distinction between amateur and professional but that division does not matter. For be an amateur or be a professional, they both are competing for the glory of winning. And hence to say that there will be no doping in Dance sport is to live in fool's paradise.[68] As the cases analyzed above reveal Dance sport is not oblivious to doping. The effectiveness of WDSF in catching the cheats in a different ball game altogether. However, to give credit to WDSF, it still has shown some interest in dealing with doping unlike many other Non-Olympic sports. Its website is better maintained considering that as a Non-Olympic sport its rigor is less. However, it also has the advantage of a Non-Olympic sport for it does not get acted against by IOC and WADA as in the case of Olympic sport. There is though one instance of WADA taking up cudgels against WDSF. This case though is the only case so far where WADA challenged the anti-doping measures of WDSF. This can be seen as both positive and negative. The positive side is that WADA can if it wants go after the Non-Olympic sport and get them to comply with the WADA Code. The negative side is that once in a while shaking up a Non-Olympic sport for compliance failure really does not take the narrative further.

In *World Anti-Doping Agency (WADA) v. International DanceSport Federation (IDSF) & Boris Maltsev & Zarina Shamsutdinova,*[69] the case decided by the WDSF Council was challenged by WADA before CAS. As noted above, the Council had reduced the ineligibility period to one year for No Significant Fault or Negligence.[70] WADA's contention was that the athletes clearly refused the dope control test. Hence, there cannot be a ground for reducing the ineligibility period to one year. WDSF (formerly IDSF) contented that "since it was a small federation with less means than some, the level of awareness of competing athletes regarding applicable rules might be inferior, which should lead to more indulgence when examining their required degree of diligence."[71] However, CAS rejected this reasoning on the ground that the WADA Code does not take into account such distinction. It is indeed problematic to argue on this line since that would bring in subjectivity in the application of the WADA Code. Further, that will lead to differential treatment among the players/athletes. CAS referred to the objective of the WADA Code, viz., to harmonize the application of the Code across different sports.[72] That precisely is the argument of the book as well. As there cannot be an argument of differential treatment based on the size of the IF, similarly there cannot be differential treatment based on the status of the sport. Thus, Olympic and Non-Olympic sports ought to be equally diligent in their compliance with the WADA Code.

CAS further harped on the point that doping is against the spirit of sport.[73] CAS then revisited the arguments that the athletes had given to the WDSF Council. As noted by CAS, the athletes argued that they have not signed "IDSF Consent Form (or other documents) accepting to submit to doping tests, that they were not warned that controls could be made and that no representative of [their federation] was present to assist them."[74] CAS rejects these contentions of the athlete since it is not mandated by the WADA Code. On the signing of the consent form, CAS notes that where the

> "[a]thletes are presented with a Form of Consent, it is mandatory for them to sign it. . ., but if none is presented to the Athlete, it cannot be mandatory to sign one . . . the absence of a Form of Consent does not relieve athletes from the obligation to abide by anti-doping rules.[75]

CAS goes onto justify this reasoning by noting that "participation in a competition necessarily implies the acceptance of the substantive rules governing the competition."[76] Explaining the absurdity that will result if this principle deviates from CAS explains that "Any other solution would lead to the absurd situation in which an athlete who participated in a competition without expressly accepting the applicable regulations by means of a signed consent form could claim all the rights of a competitor."[77] Accordingly, CAS held that

> In other words, athletes cannot be deemed to have the right to pick and choose the rules they abide by when seeking to participate in a competition. On the contrary, they must carefully inform themselves regarding the content of applicable regulations.

Accordingly, CAS held that

> the duty to submit to in-competition doping controls, are no exception, since they very much partake in establishing a level playing field in sports competitions. The existence of in-competition doping controls of elite athletes in international competitions and the duty to undergo such doping controls if one participates in those.[78]

CAS further noted that under the Anti-Doping Code of the WDSF (formerly IDSF) the "the strict obligation for all athletes who participate in competitions to accept doping-control tests is made clear in the formulation of a number of provisions"[79] Reiterating that consent can be implied and not express CAS held that

> the absence of a Consent Form cannot be deemed a valid excuse in itself, since despite the lack of such forms the Athletes decided to participate in the competition and must thereby be deemed to have accepted the competition rules.[80]

This is a very relevant point in understanding the requirements for WADA Code compliance. The idea built in is that the athletes are not forced to participate. Hence, when they do participate in a competition they are expected to be aware of the rules of their Federation or the competition. One can critique it but the present system is geared toward an approach of one-size fits all. By allowing the athletes to take up such argument and thus plead No Significant Fault or Negligence, the Non-Olympic IFs will be diluting the efficacy of the WADA Code. They will encourage their athletes to take advantage of the technical flaw and escape. CAS then went onto analyze the justification given for the reduction of the sanction.

CAS noted that "although it is not denied that both the organizers and the KDSF did not implement their respective obligations under the Anti-Doping rules, these are separate faults and do not alleviate the Athletes significant fault or negligence."[81] CAS further notes that

> the IDSF Disciplinary Committee also took into account the excuses sent by the two Athletes Panel wants to emphasize that presenting excuses after the facts cannot be considered as a mitigating factor of the violation consisting in the refusal to undergo the doping test.[82]

Accordingly, CAS held that

> As there are no elements, which can be deemed mitigating factors, the Panel finds that in the circumstances of this case as evidenced by the written documents on record, the Athletes were significantly negligent in refusing to undergo the test.[83]

This beautifully sums up the argument that one has been giving throughout, viz., laxity in WADA Code compliance on the part of the Non-Olympic sport. And the case appealed herein by WADA is shown to be a perfect example of such laxity. The outcome was that CAS reversed the decision of the WDSF Council and imposed an ineligibility period of 2 years. This is so in the absence of any mitigating factor.[84] The second case involved an appeal filed by the player against the decision of WDSF (formerly IDSF). In *D. v/ International DanceSport Federation,*[85] the athlete challenged the ineligibility period imposed by the WDSF Council on her. This is the Edita Daniute that we had discussed earlier, wherein the Council had reduced the ineligibility period to 3 months on the ground of No Significant Fault or Negligence.[86] Before the case, the athlete raised arguments of procedural unfairness and bias and conflict of interest. CAS dismissed these and observed that

> The members of disciplinary commissions of . . . sports federation are in fact . . . appointed by other bodies of the same federation: disciplinary proceedings, however intended to take place by paying due respect to the right to be heard of the parties involved, lead to decisions which can be imputed to the same federation.[87]

Thus, CAS dismissed the argument of conflict of interest and maintained that irrespective of the fact that the members of the disciplinary Panel may be appointed by the IF or the National Federation, it does not affect their objectivity. Accordingly, CAS held

> that reproach for the way specific disciplinary proceedings are organized should not be limited to an overall criticism about an alleged lack of independence or of a conflict of interest between the association and the associates, or the functional or organizational position of the disciplinary committee.[88]

One can say a lot on this for irrespective of the points CAS makes in favor of Panels created by the IFs or National Federation, they are bound to be influenced. There definitely is an apprehension of bias and conflict of interest. For the one framing the charge is the one adjudicating the matter in the case. This is problematic for the same can lead to exploitation of bargaining power. It can also lead to a decision usually in favor of the IF or the domestic federation. Hence, it is important that the adjudicating bodies appear to be objective and are free from any kind of biases. Hence, independence of the adjudicating body is essential to instill faith in the system. Notwithstanding the merit of the case, the concerns raised here were pertinent and continue to be so in the general context of sport. CAS then went into the question of the reasonability of the sanction imposed. CAS holds that it

> does not find the sanction imposed on the Dancer to be evidently and grossly disproportionate to the offence, taking into account all the elements of the case . . . including the duty of care which could be expected of a top-level athlete such as the Appellant.[89]

CAS further notes that

> that any deficiency in the anti-doping environment and culture within the IDSF system, even if existing, does not excuse practices contrary to rules in force and specifically accepted. Well to the contrary, the lower the degree of observance of the rules, the stronger the need of enforcement of those rules.[90]

These observations re-affirm the belief of the author that there is a huge gap in the enforcement mechanism within the Non-Olympic sport as against the Olympic sport.

Conclusion

WDSF needs to take the matter of enforcement seriously for there are problems galore. Notwithstanding the fact that it has well-maintained website, the information on compliance is absolutely basic. Empirical studies done by researchers in the field of Dance sport and performance-enhancing drugs have found surprising information. It was found that substance abuse is most common among the athletes in Dance sports. The research found that the athletes rarely trust their coaches or physicians in the matter of doping. It was also found that female and young athletes are more prone to doping. It was also found that anti-doping education among the athletes involved in Dance sport is poor.[91] These factors are some of many issues which WDSF needs to take note of before it aims to become an Olympic sport. Being one of the oldest Non-Olympic sport it should have set its house in order. However, till date, there are problems with respect to compliance with the WADA Code. Though the decisions delivered post 2015 appear to be better reasoned, it really does not help improve the argument of poor compliance. There is more than enough evidence that Dance sport like all others is prone to excessive doping. Dancers too need to boost stamina, heal injuries, and increase the level of oxygen in their blood. They would need better genes to increase flexibility and agility in their body. They would need to improve their concentration. They would need to increase their power and boost their physique. In short, Dancers would need all that any other athlete would need.[92] Hence, WDSF cannot push the issue of doping under the carpet. It needs to up the ante for its members and ensure that they enforce the WADA Code most stringently. It needs to improve the anti-doping education and ensure that the elite-level player does not take medication without consulting qualified practitioners.

To treat Dance differently because it is an art as well as to create a false sense of confidence. Dance may be art as well but an artist too can dope. Hence, the fact that art is also a sport and the WDSF is a signatory to WADA is a good enough reason to take doping seriously. The health reason of the athletes is a compelling issue as well for WDSF to take measures to check doping. Taking the athlete into confidence and constantly taking their feedback is needed to identify the loopholes in the compliance mechanism. Herein, WDSF needs to be pressurized by IOC and WADA. As stated again and again, the entire check and balance need to be done at the stage of granting recognition. Once the recognition is granted then the monitoring needs to be done diligently. Here IOC needs to be proactive and seeks a report from the WDSF as to the measures taken to comply with the WADA Code. In addition, WADA too needs to play a proactive role in ensuring that the WDSF does not end up letting its athlete go scot-free. WDSF's website reveals tremendous growth and popularity of the sport. Hence, to argue that it is a small IF and hence has limited resources is not convincing. Importantly, WDSF can collaborate with WADA and IOC and discharge effectively its role as the enforcer of the WADA Code. Being a Non-Olympic sport and part of the Olympic system for a long WDSF should understand the nuances of the anti-doping system. Being lax with the compliance WDSF is also putting the players at risk of getting caught. It also will mean that the players are at the risk of losing their careers. Hence, as a Non-Olympic sport with the ambition of getting admitted to the Olympic Games, it needs to be serious about compliances with the WADA Code. However, the most important role needs to be played by IOC and WADA in ensuring compliances of Non-Olympic sports.

Notes

1. Alīna Kļonova, "Partners' Physiological Engagement and Body Contact Improvement in Standard Sport Dances" www.lspa.eu/files/students/Promotion/Alina_Klonova_Promocijas_darbs.pdf (accessed 25th February 2021)
2. Ibid para 21
3. Ibid para 22
4. Ibid
5. Ibid
6. World Dance Sport Federation, "History" www.worlddancesport.org/WDSF/History (accessed 24th February 2021)
7. Global Association of International Sports Federation (GAISF), "Mission and Vision" https://gaisf.sport/mission-and-vision/ (accessed 24th February 2021)
8. World Dance Sport Federation (n 6)
9. The World Games, "The Association" www.theworldgames.org/contents/The-IWGA-15/History-of-the-IWGA-2 (accessed 24th February 2021)
10. World Dance Sport Federation (n 6)
11. Ibid
12. Ibid
13. World Dance Sport Federation, "WDSF Members" www.worlddancesport.org/WDSF/Membership (accessed 24th February 2021)
14. World Dance Sport Federation (n 6)
15. International Olympic Committee, "Olympic Charter-In Force as from 15th June 1995" https://stillmedab.olympic.org/media/Document%20Library/OlympicOrg/Olympic-Studies-Centre/List-of-Resources/Official-Publications/Olympic-Charters/EN-1995-Olympic-Charter.pdf#_ga=2.96706716.246563998.1617057514-1362183814.1617057514
16. Ibid [Chapter 3 The International Federations IFs [- Rule] 29 • Recognition of the IFs—In order to promote the Olympic Movement, the IOC may recognize as IFs international non-governmental organizations administering one or several sports at world level and encompassing organizations administering such sports at national level. The recognition of IFs newly recognized by the IOC shall be provisional for a period of two years or any other period fixed by the IOC Executive Board. At the end of such period, the recognition shall automatically lapse in the absence of definitive confirmation given in writing by the IOC. As far as the role of the IFs within the Olympic Movement is concerned, their statutes, practices, and activities must be in conformity with the Olympic Charter. Subject to the foregoing, each IF maintains its independence and autonomy in the administration of its sport.]
17. Ibid
18. Ibid [Rule 52—Sports Programme, Admission of Sports, Disciplines and Events—The IOC establishes the programme of the Olympic Games, which only includes Olympic Sports—1 Olympic Sports included in the Programme of the Olympic Games—1.1 To be included in the programme of the Olympic Games, an Olympic sport must conform to the following criteria: 1.1.1 only sports widely practised by men in at least seventy-five countries and on four continents, and by women in at least forty countries and on three continents, may be included in the programme of the Games ol the Olympiad; 1.1.2 only sports widely practised in at least twenty-five countries and on three continents may be included in the programme of the Olympic Winter Games; 1.1.3 sports are admitted to the programme of the Olympic

Games at least seven years before specific Olympic Games in respect of which no change shall thereafter be permitted.]

19. Fékou Kidane, "The 106th IOC Session" https://library.olympic.org/Default/doc/SYRACUSE/353005/the-106th-ioc-session-by-fekou-kidane (accessed 24th February 2021)
20. Ibid p 8
21. Ibid
22. Ibid
23. Jeremy Whittle, "Twenty Years on the Festina Affair Casts Shadow Over the Tour de France" www.theguardian.com/sport/2018/jul/03/tour-de-france-festina-affair (accessed 24th February 2021)
24. Ibid
25. Lovely Dasgupta, *The World Anti-Doping Code-Fit for Purpose?* (Routledge, 2019)
26. World Dance Sport Federation, "WDSF Rules and Regulations" www.worlddancesport.org/Rule/All (accessed 24th February 2021)
27. Ibid ["Anti-Doping Code-Version 1.2"]
28. Ibid p 3
29. Ibid p 4
30. World Dance Sport Federation (n 26) [WDSF Statutes] [Article 5 Admission and Termination of Membership- . . . 4. Admission to membership, and renewal of membership by payment of the annual Membership fee, constitutes a contract between the WDSF and the Member. The terms of that contract include the term that in return for membership in WDSF, Members agree to abide by the WDSF's Statutes, rules, and regulations, and to abide by decisions of the WDSF's General Meeting and Presidium, and to comply with the World Anti-Doping Code, the WDSF Anti-Doping Code, including requiring all athletes and support personnel within their jurisdiction to recognize and be bound by the World Anti-Doping Code and the WDSF Anti-Doping Code. 5. All members must be notified in writing of any new admission and of any change in membership and any change in the WDSF Professional Division. It is a condition of membership of the WDSF that the policies, rules, statutes and programs of the member comply with World Anti-Doping Code (WADC) . . .]
31. Ibid [Article 21 Rules and Regulations 1. The WDSF has the following Rules and Regulations: a) Financial Regulations b) Competition Rules c) Professional Division Rules d) Rules for Adjudication e) Regulations for Television, Broadcasting, New Media, Advertising and Sponsorship f) Anti-Doping Code g) Disciplinary Council Code h) Code of Ethics i) Code of the Ethics Committee 2. The Anti-Doping Code and the Disciplinary Council Code, the Code of Ethics and the Code of the Ethics Committee are integral parts of the Statutes.]
32. World Dance Sport Federation (n 26) ["Anti-Doping Code-Version 1.2"] [2. Anti-Doping Rule Violations- . . . 2.1 Presence of a Prohibited Substance or its Metabolites or Markers in an Athlete's Sample 2.1.1 It is the Athletes' personal duty to ensure that no Prohibited Substance enters their bodies. Athletes are responsible for any Prohibited Substance or its Metabolites or Markers found to be present in their Samples. Accordingly, it is not necessary that intent, Fault, negligence or knowing Use on the Athlete's part be demonstrated in order to establish an anti-doping rule violation under Article 2.1.]
33. World Dance Sport Federation (n 26) ["Anti-Doping Code-Version 1.2"] [3. Proof of Doping 3.1 Burdens and Standards of Proof WDSF shall have the burden of establishing that an anti-doping rule violation has occurred. The standard of proof shall be whether WDSF has established an anti-doping rule violation to the comfortable satisfaction of the hearing panel bearing in mind the seriousness of the

allegation which is made. This standard of proof in all cases is greater than a mere balance of probability but less than proof beyond a reasonable doubt. Where these Anti-Doping Rules place the burden of proof upon the Athlete or other Person alleged to have committed an anti-doping rule violation to rebut a presumption or establish specified facts or circumstances, except as provided in Articles 3.2.2 and 3.2.3, the standard of proof shall be by a balance of probability]

34. Ibid [4.2 Prohibited Substances and Prohibited Methods Identified on the Prohibited List]
35. Ibid
36. Ibid
37. World Dance Sport Federation, "WDSF PD Rules & Regulations" www.world dancesport.org/Division/Professional/Rules_and_Regulations (accessed 25th February 2021)
38. WDSF Disciplinary Council, "The Court for Dancesport" www.worlddancesport.org/WDSF/Organisation/WDSF_Disciplinary_Council (accessed 25th February 2021)
39. Ibid [IDSF Disciplinary Council Formal Decision as of 17 November 2006 regarding Violation of the IDSF Anti-Doping Code by Edita Daniute]
40. Ibid para 4.30
41. Ibid para 4.38
42. Ibid para 4.41
43. WDSF Disciplinary Council (n 38) [IDSF Disciplinary Council Formal Decision as of 3 July 2007 Regarding Alleged Violation of the IDSF Anti-Doping Code by Ivan Novikov]
44. Ibid [IDSF Disciplinary Council Formal Decision as of 3 June 2009 Regarding Violation of the IDSF Anti-Doping Code by Boris Maltsev and Zarina Shamsutdinova]
45. Ibid para 2.9–2.10
46. WDSF Disciplinary Council (n 38) [IDSF Disciplinary Council Procedural Decision as of 21th February 2011 Regarding Violation of the IDSF Anti-Doping Code by Schrebrina, Olga]
47. Ibid para 4.6
48. Ibid para 4.22
49. Ibid para 4.28
50. WDSF Disciplinary Council (n 38) [Formal Decision as of 15 July 2014 Regarding the Charge of a Violation of the WDSF Anti-Doping Code by Flora Bouchereau]
51. Ibid para 5.4
52. Ibid para 5.5
53. Ibid
54. Ibid 5.11
55. WDSF Disciplinary Council (n 38) [Formal Decision as of 29 July 2016 Regarding the Charge of a Violation of the WDSF Anti-Doping Code by Elizaveta Yuryevna Cherevichnaya]
56. WDSF Discip3.7linary Council (n 38) [Formal Decision as of 29 July 2016 Regarding the Charge of a Violation of the WDSF Anti-Doping Code by Elizaveta Yuryevna Cherevichnaya] para 5.1.2
57. Ibid para 6.2
58. Ibid para 6.10
59. Ibid para 6.11
60. WDSF Disciplinary Council (n 38) [Formal Decision as of 14 January 2018 Pertaining to a Notice of Charge for Violation of the WDSF Anti-Doping Code (ADRV) by Vitaly Panteleev and Angelina Nechkhaeva]
61. Ibid para 2.1.3
62. Ibid para 2.3.7

63. Ibid para 2.5.5
64. World Anti-Doping Agency, "World Anti-Doping Code 2015" [Article 10.2.2 If Article 10.2.1 does not apply, the period of Ineligibility shall be two years.]
65. Emily O'Neil, "Dance Is a Sport and Should Be Seen as One" https://lancasteron line.com/opinion/columnists/dance-is-a-sport-and-should-be-seen-as-one/article_ efd16800-009e-11ea-97ab-9bce5a3f99bc.html#:~:text=Dance%20is%20not%20 just%20an,another%20or%20others%20for%20entertainment.%E2%80%9D (accessed 25th February 2021)
66. Catherine Ellis, "Dance as Sport: Living Art and Commentary on the Lives of Dancers in French Literature" https://uknowledge.uky.edu/cgi/viewcontent.cgi?ar ticle=1020&context=honprog (accessed 25th February 2021)
67. Mark Dyreson, "Sport" https://science.jrank.org/pages/11323/Sport-Sport-Modern-Cultures.html (accessed 25th February 2021)
68. Blanca Rodríguez López, "Performance Enhancement and the Spirit of the Dance: Non Zero Sum" file:///C:/Users/LOVELY%20DAS%20GUPTA/Downloads/philosophies-05-00046.pdf (accessed 25th February 2021)
69. CAS 2009/A/1898
70. IDSF Disciplinary Council Formal Decision as of 3 June 2009 Regarding Violation of the IDSF Anti-Doping Code by Boris Maltsev and Zarina Shamsutdinova (n 44)
71. CAS 2009/A/1898 (n 65) para 28
72. Ibid
73. Ibid para 29
74. Ibid para 46
75. CAS 2009/A/1898 (n 65) para 52
76. Ibid para 53
77. Ibid para 54
78. Ibid para 56
79. Ibid
80. Ibid para 58
81. Ibid para 69
82. CAS 2009/A/1898 (n 65) para 70
83. Ibid para 71
84. Ibid para 72
85. CAS 2006/A/1175
86. IDSF Disciplinary Council Formal Decision as of 17 November 2006 Regarding Violation of the IDSF Anti-Doping Code by Edita Daniute (n 39)
87. CAS 2006/A/1175 para 25
88. CAS 2006/A/1175 (87) para 25
89. Ibid para 49
90. Ibid para 51
91. Damir Sekulic, Radmila Kostic and Durdica Miletic, "Substance Use in Dance Sport" www.kifst.unist.hr/~dado/index_files/MPPA2008.pdf (accessed 25th February 2021)
92. López (n 68)

References

• Alīna Kļonova, "Partners' Physiological Engagement and Body Contact Improvement in Standard Sport Dances" www.lspa.eu/files/students/Promotion/Alina_Klo nova_Promocijas_darbs.pdf (accessed 25th February 2021)
• World Dance Sport Federation, "History" www.worlddancesport.org/WDSF/History (accessed 24th February 2021)

- Global Association of International Sports Federation (GAISF), "Mission and Vision" https://gaisf.sport/mission-and-vision/ (accessed 24th February 2021)
- The World Games, "The Association" www.theworldgames.org/contents/The-IWGA-15/History-of-the-IWGA-2 (accessed 24th February 2021)
- World Dance Sport Federation, "WDSF Members" www.worlddancesport.org/WDSF/Membership (accessed 24th February 2021)
- International Olympic Committee, "Olympic Charter-in Force as from 15th June 1995" https://stillmedab.olympic.org/media/Document%20Library/OlympicOrg/Olym pic-Studies-Centre/List-of-Resources/Official-Publications/Olympic-Charters/EN-1995-Olympic-Charter.pdf#_ga=2.96706716.246563998.1617057514-1362183814.1617057514
- Fékou Kidane, "The 106th IOC Session" https://library.olympic.org/Default/doc/SYRACUSE/353005/the-106th-ioc-session-by-fekou-kidane (accessed 24th February 2021)
- Jeremy Whittle, "Twenty Years on the Festina Affair Casts Shadow Over the Tour de France" www.theguardian.com/sport/2018/jul/03/tour-de-france-festina-affair (accessed 24th February 2021)
- Lovely Dasgupta, *The World Anti-Doping Code-Fit for Purpose?* (Routledge, 2019)
- World Dance Sport Federation, "WDSF Rules and Regulations" www.worlddancesport.org/Rule/All (accessed 24th February 2021)
- World Dance Sport Federation, "WDSF PD Rules & Regulations" www.worlddancesport.org/Division/Professional/Rules_and_Regulations (accessed 25th February 2021)
- WDSF Disciplinary Council, "The Court for Dancesport" www.worlddancesport.org/WDSF/Organisation/WDSF_Disciplinary_Council (accessed 25th February 2021)
- Emily O'Neil, "Dance Is a Sport and Should Be Seen as One" https://lancasteronline.com/opinion/columnists/dance-is-a-sport-and-should-be-seen-as-one/article_efd16800-009e-11ea-97ab-9bce5a3f99bc.html#:~:text=Dance%20is%20not%20just%20an,another%20or%20others%20for%20entertainment.%E2%80%9D (accessed 25th February 2021)
- Catherine Ellis, "Dance as Sport: Living Art and Commentary on the Lives of Dancers in French Literature" https://uknowledge.uky.edu/cgi/viewcontent.cgi?article=1020&context=honprog (accessed 25th February 2021)
- Mark Dyreson, "Sport" https://science.jrank.org/pages/11323/Sport-Sport-Modern-Cultures.html (accessed 25th February 2021)
- Blanca Rodríguez López, "Performance Enhancement and the Spirit of the Dance: Non Zero Sum" file:///C:/Users/LOVELY%20DAS%20GUPTA/Downloads/philosophies-05-00046.pdf (accessed 25th February 2021)
- CAS 2009/A/1898
- CAS 2006/A/1175
- Damir Sekulic, Radmila Kostic and Durdica Miletic, "Substance Use in Dance Sport" www.kifst.unist.hr/~dado/index_files/MPPA2008.pdf (accessed 25th February 2021)

6 Wada Code, IOC, and Sovereignty

Introduction

The issue of Non-Olympic sport failing in their Code compliance measures is not disputed. Though the non-compliance with World Anti-Doping Agency (WADA) Code is not unique or confined to the Non-Olympic sport. However, their amenability to the jurisdiction of WADA depends upon their zeal to be part of the Olympic program. If Non-Olympic sports are content to be recognized by the International Olympic Committee (IOC), then one cannot argue that they will be Code compliant. For their target of being recognized by IOC is fulfilled. They have nothing much to achieve. The popularity of the sport within the domestic market will also determine the extent of compliance. If the sport is popular within the domestic market then there is no incentive for the Non-Olympic sport to undertake additional burden vis-à-vis Code compliance. Consequently, the relevance of any measure of compliance is effective if it is directly connected with the Olympics and its associated activities. Thus, for a Non-Olympic sport to comply with the WADA Code is purely a voluntary act. Hence, it is the responsibility of the WADA and the IOC to ensure that the level of compliance within the Non-Olympic sport is similar to the level within the Olympic sport. And that has to be done by being proactive vis-à-vis the Non-Olympic sport. This chapter, therefore, looks into the roles and responsibilities of the WADA and IOC vis-à-vis sports in general. The chapter begins by analyzing the Code monitoring responsibilities of the various stakeholder. Primarily, the WADA and IOC. It looks into the standards developed for determining compliance failure. It looks into the International Standards that are in place vis-à-vis compliance measures of the various stakeholders. It primarily focuses on the consequence of the IFs for non-compliance. This chapter then looks into the compliance enforcement efforts with respect to Non-Olympic sports. The role of WADA and IOC is especially looked into to understand the importance of the Non-Olympic sport within the framework of anti-doping regulation. This chapter also tries to investigate the rationale behind extending the Code compliance responsibilities to the State signatories. The chapter questions the rationale of bringing the State into the picture. The chapter argues that in so far as the Non-Olympic sports are concerned the State ought not to be held

DOI: 10.4324/9781003082309-6

liable. The process of recognition and de-recognition is exclusively the domain of IOC, hence States cannot be blamed for their laxities. This holds true even more for those Non-Olympic sports which do not depend on State funding. Hence, the WADA Code compliance cannot be used by IOC to usurp the sovereignty of the State. An exception ought to be made in case of Non-Olympic sport in this regard.

WADA and IOC—Setting the Stage for Code Compliance

Article 20 of the WADA Code[1] details out the roles and responsibilities of the IOC and WADA. IOC is required first and foremost to frame rules and policies that are in confirmation with the WADA Code.[2] The IOC is also responsible to ensure that International Federations (IFs) applying for recognition are Code compliant.[3] Code compliance is a condition precedent to the recognition process. In effect therefore the first entity to ensure that the IFs are in compliance with the Code is IOC.[4] If the IOC is strict with its monitoring then there will be more pressure on the IFs in terms of Code compliance. However, as was noted in the case of Dance sport, some IFs have got recognition without having to prove any robust anti-doping program.[5] For that matter, this argument applies to all the sports irrespective of their status as an Olympic or a Non-Olympic sport. One has to understand that the IOC has commercial compulsions as well hence the consideration for granting recognition is varied.[6] It may not be too far from the truth to say that the more lucrative the market is the more chance the sport has to be included in the Olympic program.[7] That IOC is important for the success of the WADA anti-doping program is evident from the clear stipulation that requires IOC to stop all kinds of financial support.[8] That financial incentives are important for sustaining the sport is evident from our discussion on the relationship of IFAF and NFL.[9] Continuing with the responsibilities of the IOC, it has to ensure that all the entities under its aegis are Code compliant.[10] That is also reiterated in Article 12 of the WADA Code.[11]

IOC has immense power to impose sanctions whenever it decides so.[12] Considering its status as the sport behemoth, there are not many IFs or even State that can mess with IOC.[13] Furthering the narrative on the responsibilities that the IOC, the Code stipulates that the IOC ought to mandate all its athletes as well as employees and other officials to strictly comply with WADA Code.[14] IOC is also expected to promote and nurture the Independent Observer Program.[15] The Independent Observer program is to enable WADA to observe the going on within the various International Sports competitions. Since most of the International sports competitions are under the aegis of the IOC or recognized by IOC, WADA's Independent Observer program depends on the cooperation of the IOC.[16] Thus, the Independent Observer can look into the anti-doping compliance by the IFs or the Organizing body of the competition. It is an important aspect to ensure the success of the anti-doping program. IOC is also required to pursue all cases of ADRV committed by athletes under its jurisdiction.[17] Hence, all the ADRV cases committed in the Olympic Games for example need to be taken up by the IOC.[18] IOC is also entrusted with the responsibility of conducting anti-doping education program for all under its jurisdiction.[19] This too is an important aspect of strengthening the WADA Code compliance. However, the most important of all the responsibilities is the requirement for IOC to select host countries based on their anti-doping compliance record.[20]

The selection of host cities/countries has been in the past primarily been dictated by commercial incentives. IOC has been criticized for its decision to award the hosting rights to countries having poor records in human rights. Though IOC denied such allegations in the past. However, an express clause within the WADA Code vis-à-vis anti-doping compliance makes it essential for IOC to abide by the same. Accordingly, IOC too has made necessary changes within its Charter to enable it to be Code compliant. Thus, IOC has added Rule 43 making WADA code compliance mandatory for the entire Olympic move-ment.[21] Importantly, IOC has made WADA Code compliance mandatory for all essential activities relating to the administration as well as running of the IOC. For instance, in Bye-Law 2.3 to Rule 16 dealing with IOC Members Elec-tion Commission, the candidature will also be evaluated on the compliance record of the candidates of the IFs or National Olympic Committee (NOC).[22] Similarly, Bye-Law 7 to Rule 21, the establishment of a Medical-Scientific Commission to ensure WADA Code compliance.[23] Similarly, the NOCs are also mandated with WADA Code compliance measures.[24] As explained earlier, IOC makes WADA Code compliance a prerequisite for participation in the Olympic Games.[25] And the requirement for WADA Code compliance has been reiterated again and again throughout the Olympic Charter.[26] Thus, IOC can impose a sanction for non-compliance, can cancel membership, and impor-tantly can remove a sport of an IF from the Olympic program. The removal from the Olympic program is a serious issue as is the issue of sanction. In both the cases, the financial incentives of being Olympic sports are getting hit. It is important that the IFs be on the right side of the law and ensure WADA Code compliance. And it is also important for the IOC to be proactive and implement these powers with proper reasoning. For the same is an important weapon in forcing the IFs to comply with the WADA Code. In effect, the existence of the WADA Code can be threatened if the IOC does not put in the requisite effort to ensure Code compliance. The Charter thus tries to bring in a harmony between the WADA Code and the IOC obligations. Unfortunately, this easier said than done.

WADA imposes further responsibilities on the IOC by requiring it to coop-erate with other anti-doping organizations for the smooth functioning and implementation of the WADA Code. In addition, the WADA Code also stipu-lates that the IOC respects the autonomy of the accredited laboratories acting under the authority and recognition of WADA. Finally, the IOC is requested to implement policies in order to facilitate the implementation of the WADA Code within the Olympic movement.[27] As we have seen, the IOC Charter has indeed incorporated stringent provisions to ensure WADA Code compliance.

However, their effectiveness will depend on the proactive approach that the IOC will take in ensuring no laxity exists in the implementation of the WADA Code. Under the WADA Code, WADA too is entrusted with the responsibilities of ensuring Code compliance.[28] As the organization in charge of the implementation of the Code understandable, the first and foremost responsibility is to accept the Code.[29] WADA is the foremost authority on whom the success of the Code depends. Hence, it has the most crucial responsibility to ensure that the recognized stakeholders do not deviate from the Code. Accordingly, it has adopted, as it is required to, policies and procedures to ensure effective implementation of the Code.[30] And one of the most important roles of the WADA is to be the facilitator of Code compliance. Thus, it is responsible to facilitate and guide the various stakeholders to implement the Code and comply effectively with its provisions.[31] WADA is also entrusted with the task of developing and approving International Standards for various aspects relating to the implementation of the Code.[32] The International Standards are necessary to further the agenda of WADA of harmonizing the anti-doping program. The International Standard does away with any arbitrary or discretionary program that the individual stakeholder might think of implementing.

WADA is also entrusted with the task of accrediting the laboratories to conduct tests and other aspects of sample collection and preservation.[33] The task accrediting is also standardized through the principles developed by WADA. Though the accreditation itself does not ensure that the lab will not tamper with results or manipulate the outcome. And that is the reason why a strong monitoring system is needed to check that the accreditation is not abused by the lab.[34] Similarly, the WADA also develops and has indeed developed models of best practice to be followed by different stakeholders.[35] Again this is effective only when there is stringent monitoring on the part of WADA. Mere framing of the best practice guidelines will hardly ensure the Code compliance. WADA in order to soften the rigor of the Code has accommodated the concerns of the athletes. Accordingly, it has the responsibility to place before its board the concerns of the athletes with respect to the protection of their rights.[36] The WADA is thus trying to bring about inclusivity in the anti-doping program. The fruitfulness of this approach and the eventual benefit to the athletes through this process is not clear. Though it is a welcome move on the part of the WADA. In pursuance of this responsibility, WADA indeed has brought in force on June 18, 2020, the Athletes' Anti-Doping Rights Act. The same was approved by the WADA's Executive Committee at the World Conference.

> The Act, which was developed by WADA's Athlete Committee in consultation with thousands of athletes and stakeholders worldwide, is based on the 2021 Code and Standards and aims to ensure that athlete rights within anti-doping are clearly set out, accessible, and universally applicable.[37]

This is an important development toward incorporating the concerns of the athlete. Importantly, from the perspective of the present discussion, it will incentivize the athletes to comply with the WADA Code.

WADA is also entrusted with the responsibility of conducting anti-doping education as well as research.[38] This is important to promote the cause of anti-doping compliance for the increase of awareness will lead the stakeholders to be cautious about their conduct. The anti-doping behavior will accordingly become more in tune with the expected behavior and not contrary to it. It is to achieve this objective that the WADA is also required to develop Independent Observer program as well as advisory programs.[39]

WADA is entrusted with the task of conducting[40] tests suo moto whenever needed. WADA can also do the same upon the request of another Anti-Doping Organization. All this is geared toward ensuring the effective compliance of the Code by the signatories. Further, the power to participate or facilitate inquiries and investigation will enable WADA to better check any manipulation done by the signatory. ADRV cases will also be better tracked and reported. However, in real terms, its effectiveness will need to be seen in the distant future. WADA is empowered to approve specific anti-doping programs involving sample testing and analysis of the data. This is done in consultation with the concerned stakeholder.[41] WADA also has the responsibility to see to it that all its members as well as employees and personnel working for WADA are Code compliant.[42] And in furtherance of this responsibility, WADA has to refrain from association with persons accused of ADRV. The persons need to be under suspension for ADRV. It can also be one who, though outside the ambit of WADA, committed ADRV. In all these cases, the WADA needs to avoid all kinds of associations with such individuals.[43] Finally, WADA has been conferred with the most important tool to deal with anti-doping violations, especially, the one which is hard to detect and can only be uncovered through investigations and intelligence gathering. The need to investigate and gather intelligence on systematic doping arose in light of the Russian doping scandal.

The stakeholders felt the need to empower WADA with the investigation and intelligence gathering authority.[44] Hence, WADA can at suspicious of doping infractions as well as violation of compliance requirement initiate investigations.[45] The aforementioned roles and responsibilities of the IOC and WADA are in addition to their existing responsibilities under the Code. The above-stated responsibilities thus only enhance the scope of the power the two bodies have. Considering that in the pyramidal structure within the world of sport IOC is the supreme authority, its decisions and conduct make an impact on the compliance with the Code.[46] Importantly, the role of IOC in promoting and propagating the importance of the WADA Code has the power to convince the IFs about effective compliance.[47] IOC has to bear the principal responsibility to ensure that the WADA Code is complied with effectively. And IOC can do the same by having a smooth coordination with WADA. Thus, the detailing out of the roles and responsibilities of the WADA and IOC is necessary. It is so because this explains the power structure that exists within the world of sports. It also identifies the efforts that the IOC and WADA ought to put in to ensure that the stakeholders comply with the WADA Code. Importantly, it helps better perceive the importance of the International standards that have been subsequently developed to outline the requirements for compliance and its monitoring. A perusal of the said document hence will be done now to further highlight the importance of compliance. Importantly, it will once again underline the fact that Non-Olympic sports have no compulsion to have a robust anti-doping system unless IOC and WADA streamline their attitude. In other words, unless the IOC and WADA show their zeal, the Non-Olympic sport will continue to evade compliance requirements with impunity.

WADA Code Compliance—The Standard and the Intent

All need to be clear that WADA is not the adjudicating body to determine the question of non-compliance. Hence, it cannot impose the consequence of non-compliance on its own. However, as per the WADA Code, power is given to the WADA to monitor and enforce compliance with the Code.[48] WADA is given the power to ask all the signatories to report compliance measures to it.[49] Any failure to submit such information or submission of incorrect information will be regarded as a violation of the Code.[50] WADA will try getting the signatory to correct its deviance from the Code and follow the procedure laid down in the International Standard For Code Compliance.[51] Any defiance by the signatory to follow the advisory of WADA will lead it to be declared as Code Non-Compliant. On the other hand, if the signatory accedes to the finding of the WADA on non-compliance, it needs to act promptly as per the decision of the WADA in the matter.[52] Any dispute raised by the signatory on the finding of the WADA about its non-compliance will have to be contested and raised before CAS. The burden placed on WADA to prove its case is the balance of probability.[53] Upon the dispute being referred to CAS WADA will issue a public notice about the said fact. The said notice is also relevant to facilitate all interested stakeholders to intervene in the matter. The entities who can intervene are IOC, IFs to be affected by the decision of CAS as well as any other person with the prior permission of CAS.[54] The decision of CAS in the dispute will be final subject to the right of appeal to the Swiss Federal Tribunal (SFT).[55] The decision of the CAS in the matter will be binding on all signatories and are to be observed by all.[56] The dispute with the signatory can also arise with respect to the reinstatement conditions. In other words, WADA can refuse to re-instate the signatory on the ground that it has yet to fulfill the conditions laid down. The signatory can take the dispute to CAS. In all cases of dispute pertaining to non-compliance, the matter will be heard by the CAS Ordinary Arbitration Division.[57] Further, the compliance requirement imposed upon the signatories varies as per the categories specified in the International Standard For Code Compliance.[58] This classification ranges from critical to high priority to general. The signatory can challenge the classification before CAS. Finally, in case of non-compliance being established, the facts and circumstances of a case will determine the kind of consequence that will be imposed on the signatory. The first and foremost consequence that may be imposed in the withdrawal of all facilities and support of WADA.[59] The signatory may also face the consequence of missing out on organization or hosting of International sporting events.[60]

The signatory misses out being part of all WADA observers or outreach programs.[61] The signatory will also lose out on all kinds of funding from WADA.[62] The representative of the signatory is barred from holding all official positions in any capacity whatsoever with any other signatories.[63] WADA will have the power to impose a continuous monitoring system on the defaulting signatory till it becomes a Code complaint.[64] The monitoring and compliance provisions of the Code also permit the takeover of the defaulting signatories' anti-doping activities.[65] Apart from these, the signatories may also be imposed with fine.[66] The defaulting signatory is also likely to lose out on funding from IOC and other IFs or Sports Organization, who is a signatory to the Code.[67] The non-compliance by the signatory also has effects beyond the field of sports. Hence, any public body finding the signatory will be required to stop such funding upon the default of the signatory on Code compliance.[68] The default on the part of the signatory will have consequences for its country which too will be barred from hosting international sports competitions.[69] And the consequences are further accentuated by the default of the signatory leading to a complete ban of the concerned country/NOC/athletes and their representatives.[70] Consequences are equally detrimental for Ifs, which have failed to comply with the Code.[71] Similarly, a Major Event Organizer also faces a ban and other severe consequences for failing to comply with the Code.[72] Importantly, from the perspective of the current discussion, the non-compliance will lead to suspension of recognition of an IF.[73] Finally, the WADA permits other signatories as well as countries to impose additional burden/sanction on the defaulting signatory.[74]

In case of decisions given by WADA and accepted by the signatory in connection with the finding of non-compliance, are appealable to CAS under Article 13.6 of the Code.[75] The provisions stipulated in Article 24.1 of the Code, as noted above are important. For they strengthen the WADA and makes monitoring and compliance more effective. One still has reservations as to its effectiveness vis-à-vis Non-Olympic sports. Nonetheless, the provisions are stringent enough to make the signatories vigilant. It is thus equally necessary to understand the scope of the International Standard for Code Compliance by Signatories (ISCCS).[76] The ISCCS outlines the objective of the standards as those relating to the implementation of harmonized, effective, and transparent anti-doping system under the Code. Accordingly, it sets out the (1) roles, responsibilities of the various entities involved in the enforcement of the WADA Code, and ensuring its compliance; (2) details out support and assistance and guidance that WADA will provide to the signatories to ensure effective compliance; (3) the monitoring system that will be used by WADA to ensure compliances; (4) the logistical support and facilities that the signatories will be provided with for course correction with respect to their compliance obligation; (5) details of the procedure to be followed before CAS; (6) principle to be followed by CAS while determining the consequences of non-compliance; (7) procedure for earliest reinstatement of the signatory found to be non-compliant, post-course correction; and (8) details the transitional provision.[77]

These standards are mandatory and provide for the norms that need to be followed to determine compliance with the Code. The essential objective is for WADA to converse with the signatories and through dialogue convince them to have strong and robust compliance systems in place. To support the signatories in a manner that they are smoothly reinstated upon course correction. For overseeing Code compliance by the signatories WADA has constituted a special task force that works with the Compliance Review Committee (CRC). Through this mechanism, WADA develops a procedure to monitor compliance, detects non-compliance, and assists signatories with course correction as well as reinstatement in the list of complaint signatories.[78] The CRC is constituted as an apolitical, independent review committee overseeing the compliance, monitoring, and enforcing efforts of WADA. It also provides advice and recommendation to the WADA Executive Committee in case any signatory fails to comply with the Code.[79] An important aspect of the ISCCS is the effort to amicably resolve issues of non-compliance by giving opportunities to the signatory for course correction. According to this theme, a course correction chance is given to the signatory even at the last stage. Hence, before the consequence for non-compliance, as determined by CAS are to be imposed, the signatory can correct the non-compliance.[80] Reinstatement criteria and the fulfillment of the same are determined by the CRC.[81] ISCCS details the support WADA is to provide to the signatories for ensuring Code compliance as well as maintaining the same.[82] In addition, ISCCS also lays down the parameter for monitoring the Code compliance efforts.[83]

One thing that is very clear is that the ISCCS also enables WADA to prioritize the efforts of ensuring compliance with the Code. The ISCCS has thus provided a list of potential factors which need to be taken into account by WADA for prioritizing the enforcement and compliance monitoring efforts.[84] The argument primarily is the limited resources at the disposal of WADA. This explains the reason why more effort is given toward monitoring the compliance issues of Olympic sport as compared to the Non-Olympic sport. And that creates the problem for then it all comes down to the compliance efforts of the individual IF. However, as reviewed above, the immense power conferred to WADA really makes it necessary that equal priority is given to Olympic as well as Non-Olympic sports. Again the argument of limited resource is used to categorize the compliance requirement as critical, high priority, or normal. The WADA expands its efforts in ensuring compliance with the critical and high priority requirements as against the normal ones. For the normal ones, signatories are given additional opportunities to comply with the normal requirements. The severest consequence is meant for the non-compliance of the critical requirements.[85] Monitoring tools used by WADA is comprehensive enough to use all tools permissible under the law. Thus, WADA can access all the documents and data legitimately to check upon the compliance level of the signatories.[86]

In addition, the signatory may be asked to provide certain mandatory information in cases where WADA is suspicious of the signatories' compliance level. Especially where the WADA has ground to believe that the signatory is evading complying with the critical and high priority requirements.[87] To further the task of effective monitoring of the compliance efforts of the signatories, WADA in consultation with the CRC conduct a Compliance Audit selectively. It will choose the signatory under this Compliance Audit.[88] Again with respect to continuous monitoring of the compliance by signatories, WADA will consult the CRC.[89] Again this will be done selectively. Such selective monitoring is again justified by the limited resource argument that WADA has codified through the ISCCS. This selective monitoring is problematic at two levels. At the first level, it is problematic because it might not be applied to low-key sport and small federations lacking high-profile athlete or fan base. Second, it is problematic from the perspective of Non-Olympic sport because they would largely be ignored unless they fit the bill of a high-profile sport. The ISCCS also spells out the criteria to be used to determine compliances by the Major Sports Event Organization like the IOC. In order to fast track the course correction in respect of these Major Sports event Organization, Independent Observer program is used.[90] ISCCS also lays down the procedure for giving an opportunity to the signatories for course correction.[91]

CRC comes in only when signatories continue to refuse course correction and dispute the claim of WADA vis-à-vis non-compliance. CRC, after considering all the facts, will recommend according to the WADA Executive Committee.[92] The CRC will accordingly recommend sending a formal notice to the signatory of non-compliance and the nature of requirement not complied with.[93] It is up to the WADA Executive Committee to accept or reject or partially accept the recommendation of the CRC and act accordingly.[94] The signatories too have the option of accepting the decision of non-compliance or raise the dispute before CAS.[95] However, as noted above the principle of last resort is applied and even at the stage of implementing the decision of CAS, the signatory can go for course correction. In that case, the consequences are not imposed.[96]

ISCCS also specifies the principles that ought to be kept in mind while imposing the consequence of non-compliance on the signatory. The consequence needs to be in proportion with the nature of the non-compliance and the degree of fault of the signatory. Similarly, if there are aggravating factors, the consequence will be severe. The application of the consequence will be without discrimination and fair. Hence, the consequence imposed cannot be greater than what is necessary in view of the fault/non-compliance. Imposition of the consequence should be such as to give rise to confidence in the process among the parties. The effect of the consequence should lead to cessation of all activities in non-compliance with the Code. The consequence will become severe if the signatory fails to satisfy the reinstatement criteria.[97] The criteria for being reinstated are also detailed out in the ISCCS. And the objective is to smoothly complete the process of reinstatement without compromising on the objective of enforcing compliance. The WADA will issue a public notice once the reinstatement process is successfully completed.[98]

Thus, ISCCS forms an important document in ensuring compliances with the WADA Code. The ISCCS along with the provisions of the Code, as referred above can equally be used to ensure compliance in the case of Non-Olympic sports. This is necessary to override the existing disparity between Olympic and Non-Olympic sports. It is necessary to harmonize the implementation of WADA across all sports. It is needed for the lack of focus on Non-Olympic sport will make the whole exercise of designing compliance standards futile. WADA cannot rely on limited resources to ignore Non-Olympic sports. It is needed precisely for the very reason that WADA Code exists. WADA Code emphatically declares that its purpose is to protect the

> Athletes' fundamental right to participate in doping-free sport and thus promote health, fairness and equality for Athletes worldwide, and • To ensure harmonized, coordinated and effective anti-doping programs at the international and national level with regard to the prevention of doping. . . .[99]

Hence, ignoring the situation within Non-Olympic sports is to breach this fundamental and core principle of WADA. The lack of their participation within the Olympic Games should be a good reason enough to scrutinize the compliance level of Non-Olympic sports. Importantly, by not being proactive in the case of Non-Olympic sports, one is essentially making a mockery of the principle of non-discrimination and fairness. That compliance with the Code is poor among the Non-Olympic sport can be gauged from the ADRV cases actually reported or decided. Another troubling issue is the failure of Non-Olympic sports to comply with the Code can put their countries into trouble.

Compliance Mess Among Non-Olympic Sports—A State in Trouble

As per the 2018 ADRV Report submitted by WADA, the number of samples tested by the Non-Olympic sport is 13,129 and resulted in 110 ADRV.[100] Considering that the Association of IOC Recognized International Sports Federations (ARISF) has 40-odd-member IFs, the number of samples tested is not encouraging. In contrast, the Association of Summer Olympics International Federations (ASOIF) has 25-odd members. And as per the report, the number of samples tested by ASOIF is 1,99,602 leading to 955 ADRV.[101] This is an important parameter to gather the state of affairs among Non-Olympic sports. Now, it is a fact that the Non-Olympic sports are signatories to the WADA Code. Having gone through Article 24.1.12.9 of the Code[102] as well as the

ISCCS,[103] the consequences for non-compliance are severe. It goes to the extent of banning the country and depriving the country of hosting all kinds of international sports competitions. In the case of a Non-Olympic sport IF, the trouble will be at two levels. One will be at the level of the IF itself. Being a signatory its failure to comply with the WADA Code will attract consequences as mentioned in Article 24.1.12 as well as the ISCCS. The Non-Olympic sport will, as mentioned, lose its status of recognized sports. And that will definitely affect its sustainability as a sport. The schemes and programs that such an IF have been promoting or designing will equally lose their steam. Primarily because getting recognized by IOC is a big financial boost to a sport at the International level. Hence, it is in the interest of the IFs that it takes care of the compliance.

However, as seen in the case of Non-Olympic sports discussed herein, the compliance can only be possible if the WADA, using its power, nudges them. IFs can always argue that there are not many reported cases of ADRVs in Non-Olympic sports. However, that will not suffice for the day they are caught flouting the Code the outcome will be serious. As can be seen in the case of *World Anti-Doping Agency v. Russian Anti-Doping Agency.*[104] Russia too got caught unawares and its Code violations have been well documented. The case was another in the series of multiple disputes involving the Russian athletes and their agencies. In this case, CAS had to look into the Code violations committed by the Russian Agency. Especially in view of the plea of the Russian Agency to be reinstated in the list of Code compliant signatories. CAS went through the detailed arguments given on both sides and held that

> The Russian Anti-Doping Agency ("RUSADA") is found to be non-compliant with the World Anti-Doping Code ("WADC") in connection with its failure to procure that the authentic LIMS data and underlying analytical data of the former Moscow Laboratory was received by WADA.[105]

CAS found that "RUSADA failed to comply with the Post-Reinstatement Data Requirement, this Panel has accordingly imposed consequences to reflect the nature and seriousness of the non-compliance and to ensure that the integrity of sport against the scourge of doping is maintained."[106] This is quite relevant for the Non-Olympic sports who are conveniently being lax about Code compliance. Considering that till date, the IFs have not been brought to the book really cannot lull them to sleep. The Non-Olympic sport needs to be more proactive about their compliance measures. They can start by testing samples on a larger scale and duly reporting the cases of ADRV. WADA's role in forcing the Non-Olympic IFs to comply with the Code will also help them avoid the consequences of non-compliance, as referred above. The case of *Andrea Iannone v. FIM and WADA v. FIM and Andrea Iannone*[107] is an example of the role that WADA can play. Mr. Andrea Iannone, a professional motorcycle racer, was charged with ADRV. The ADRV was caused due to the

presence of Drostanolone a prohibited substance and is an Anabolic Andro-
genic Steroids (AAS).[108]

The athlete was found to have No Significant Fault or Negligence and his
ineligibility period was reduced to 18 months. Before CAS WADA challenged this finding. The athlete also challenged the finding on the ground that
the ineligibility period is excessive. WADA contends that this was a case of
intentional doping hence there should not be any reduction in the ineligibility period. CAS after going through the arguments and counter-arguments of
all the sides noted that the standard four-year period of ineligibility[109] could
be avoided by the athlete either by showing a lack of intent based on concrete and persuasive evidence on a balance of probabilities or by showing
that "such period should be reduced based on no significant fault or negligence."[110] Accordingly, CAS notes that the athlete has not proven a lack of
intention on the balance of probability.[111] And that was good enough to reverse
the decision of FIM and uphold the contention of WADA. CAS thus declares
that "Mr. Iannone has not been able to meet his burden of proof to establish the same on a balance of probabilities for purposes of establishing that
the ADVR that he committed was unintentional pursuant to Article 10.2 of
ADC."[112] Accordingly, the ineligibility period that was applied was the standard 4 years. The case is again a testimony to the fact that the Non-Olympic
IFs are lax in their Code compliance. Importantly, they give excessive leeway
to their athletes. They are not stringent in their analyses of the evidence or the
arguments that the athletes put up to explain their ADRV. Non-Olympic IFs
are ready to reduce the ineligibility period without any clear proof of innocence or other mitigating factors. Thus, WADA has to intervene and ensure
that they apply the Code as it is meant to be and not as per the whims of the
Non-Olympic sports IF.

The second level at which there might be a problem is for a State in the
context of laxity in compliance by the Non-Olympic sports. It is a fact that
the signatories to the Code are all part of the Olympic movement and it does
not involve governments. However, the National Anti-Doping Agencies are
usually established by the Government of the concerned country. Additionally, almost all the governments have committed themselves to anti-doping
measures by signing the Copenhagen Declaration on Anti-Doping in Sport of
March 3, 2003.[113] This led to the signing and ratification of the UNESCO Anti-
Doping Convention by almost all the governments of the world.[114] Hence, there
is an obligation on the Countries to ensure that the signatories under their jurisdiction comply with the WADA Code. In the context of Non-Olympic sports, if
there is laxity at the level of both the IF and its member, the consequence will
have to be faced by the State. The States will be sidelined and treated as outcast
if the Non-Olympic sports are proven to be flouting the Code. One should learn
from the example of Russia and the consequence it faced. Though that might
be an extreme situation, however, the States cannot escape their liability due to
laxity on the part of the Non-Olympic sports. For the consequence will be the
same be it Olympic or Non-Olympic sport. This is evident from Article 22 of

the WADA Code. It clearly mentions the consequences that the State will bear in case of the signatories within its jurisdiction do not comply with the Code.[115] Further Article 24 also mentions the consequence that the State may have to bear in case of default of the signatories, under its jurisdiction, to comply with the Code.[116]

Conclusion

The Non-Olympic sports are the creation of the IOC. The recognition is granted by the IOC; hence, the liability to ensure Code compliance has to be on the IOC. Considering the excessive power that the Code has conferred on WADA, it too is equally responsible for the non-compliance of the Non-Olympic sports. In this setup, the State is just a bystander more so in a situation where the State has not contributed to the non-compliance. The Non-Olympic sports, not being part of the Olympic movement, do not make the State realize their obligations under the WADA Code. Importantly, the State can only be made liable where it has aided or abetted systemic doping. The State thus should be held liable when it has explicitly gone back in its commitment under the UNESCO Convention. And that should be limited to the Olympic sports for the State definitely has the duty to ensure that the IFs participating in the Olympic program and IOC-recognized event are Code compliant. Importantly, since they are being sent on behalf of the National Olympic Committees that use the color and flag of the concerned State. In case of Non-Olympic sports, such participation within the Olympic movement is missing. The Non-Olympic sports are primarily confined to the competitions that their IFs. They may participate in multisport competitions where Non-Olympic sport IF is a member. This clear demarcation between the status of Olympic sport as compared to Non-Olympic sport is a ground that the States should be exempted. A Non-Olympic sport exemption ought to be created in favor of the State within the Code. As the State is not responsible if IOC and WADA, without applying any rigor, grant recognition to all and sundry. Any arm twisting in this regard of the State will be usurping their Sovereignty. The State should also not be liable in the case of those sports that do not depend on State funding for their existence. In such a case even if the State allows its flag and logo to be used by such a sport it still does not bear responsibility. For the conduct is exclusive of the sport concerned and being a Code signatory they ought to on their own comply with WADA.

Notes

1. World Anti-Doping Agency, "World Anti-Doping Code 2021" [Article 20 Additional Roles and Responsibilities of Signatories and WADA Each Anti-Doping Organization may delegate aspects of Doping Control or anti-doping Education for which it is responsible but remains fully responsible for ensuring that any aspect it delegates is performed in compliance with the Code. To the extent such delegation is made to a Delegated Third Party that is not a Signatory, the agreement with the

Delegated Third Party shall require its compliance with the Code and International Standards.]

2. Ibid [20.1 Roles and Responsibilities of the International Olympic Committee 20.1.1 to Adopt and Implement Anti-Doping Policies and Rules for the Olympic Games which Conform with the Code and the International Standards.]

3. Ibid [20.1.2 To Require, as a Condition of Recognition by the International Olympic Committee, That International Federations and National Olympic Committees Within the Olympic Movement are in Compliance with the Code and the International Standards.]

4. International Olympic Committee, "Olympic Charter - In Force as from 17 July 2020" [25 Recognition of IFs. In order to develop and promote the Olympic Movement, the IOC may recognise as IFs international non-governmental organisations governing one or several sports at the world level, which extends by reference to those organisations recognised by the IFs as governing such sports at the national level. The statutes, practice and activities of the IFs within the Olympic Movement must be in conformity with the Olympic Charter, including the adoption and implementation of the World Anti-Doping Code as well as the Olympic Movement Code on the Prevention of Manipulation of Competitions. Subject to the foregoing, each IF maintains its independence and autonomy in the governance of its sport.]

5. See Chapter 5

6. Richard Pound, "The Olympics and the Paradox of Commercialization" https://hbr.org/2012/08/the-olympics-and-the-paradox-o (accessed 25th February 2021)

7. Mark P. Lagon and Katharine Nasielski, "Tarnished Gold: Human Rights Violations and World Sport" https://freedomhouse.org/article/tarnished-gold-human-rights-violations-and-world-sport (accessed 25th February 2021)

8. World Anti-Doping Agency (n 1) [20.1.3 To withhold some or all Olympic funding and/ or other benefits from sport organizations that are not in compliance with the Code and/or the International Standards, where required under Article 24.1.]

9. See Chapter 3

10. World Anti-Doping Agency (n 1) [20.1.4 To take appropriate action to discourage noncompliance with the Code and the International Standards (a) by Signatories, in accordance with Article 24.1 and the International Standard for Code Compliance by Signatories, and (b) by any other sporting body over which it has authority, in accordance with Article 12.]

11. Ibid [Article 12 Sanctions by Signatories Against Other Sporting Bodies Each Signatory shall adopt rules that obligate each of its member organizations and any other sporting body over which it has authority to comply with, implement, uphold and enforce the Code within that organization's or body's area of competence. When a Signatory becomes aware that one of its member organizations or other sporting body over which it has authority has failed to fulfill such obligation, the Signatory shall take appropriate action against such organization or body. In particular, a Signatory's action and rules shall include the possibility of excluding all, or some group of, members of that organization or body from specified future Events or all Events conducted within a specified period of time.]

12. Travis Nelson, "Sport Without Referees? The Power of the International Olympic Committee and the Social Politics of Accountability" www.icsspe.org/system/files/Nelson%20%26%20Cottrell%20-%20Sport%20without%20referees%20-%20The%20power%20of%20the%20IOC%20and%20the%20social%20politiscs%20of%20accountability.pdf (accessed 25th February 2021)

13. Jonathan Grix and Donna Lee, "Soft Power, Sports Mega-Events and Emerging States: The Lure of the Politics of Attraction" www.tandfonline.com/doi/pdf/10.1080/13600826.2013.827632 (accessed 25th February 2021)

14. World Anti-Doping Agency (n 1) [20.1.6 To require all Athletes preparing for or participating in the Olympic Games, and all Athlete Support Personnel associated with such Athletes, to agree to and be bound by anti-doping rules in conformity with the Code as a condition of such participation or involvement. 20.1.7 Subject to applicable law, as a condition of such position or involvement, to require all of its board members, directors, officers, and those employees (and those of appointed Delegated Third Parties), who are involved in any aspect of Doping Control, to agree to be bound by antidoping rules as Persons in conformity with the Code for direct and intentional misconduct, or to be bound by comparable rules and regulations put in place by the Signatory. 20.1.8 Subject to applicable law, to not knowingly employ a Person in any position involving Doping Control (other than authorized anti-doping Education or rehabilitation programs) who is Provisionally Suspended or is serving a period of Ineligibility under the Code or, if a Person was not subject to the Code, who has directly and intentionally engaged in conduct within the previous six (6) years which would have constituted a violation of anti-doping rules if Code-compliant rules had been applicable to such Person.]
15. Ibid [20.1.5 To authorize and facilitate the Independent Observer Program]
16. World Anti-Doping Agency, "Independent Observer Program" www.wada-ama. org/en/what-we-do/independent-observer-program (accessed 25th February 2021)
17. World Anti-Doping Agency (n 1) [20.1.9 To vigorously pursue all potential anti-doping rule violations within its authority including investigation into whether Athlete Support Personnel or other Persons may have been involved in each case of doping.]
18. IOC—Greg Martin, "Pre-Games Anti-Doping Programme for Tokyo 2020 to be the Most Extensive Ever" www.olympic.org/news/pre-games-anti-doping-programme-for-tokyo-2020-to-be-the-most-extensive-ever (accessed 25th February 2021)
19. World Anti-Doping Agency (n 1) [20.1.10 To plan, implement, evaluate and promote antidoping Education in line with the requirements of the International Standard for Education.]
20. World Anti-Doping Agency (n 1) [20.1.11 To accept bids for the Olympic Games only from countries where the government has ratified, accepted, approved or acceded to the UNESCO Convention, and (where required under Article 24.1.9) to not accept bids for Events from countries where the National Olympic Committee, the National Paralympic Committee and/or the National Anti-Doping Organization is not in compliance with the Code or the International Standards.]
21. International Olympic Committee (n 4) [43 World Anti-Doping Code and the Olympic Movement Code on the Prevention of Manipulation of Competitions Compliance with the World Anti-Doping Code and the Olympic Movement Code on the Prevention of Manipulation of Competitions is mandatory for the whole Olympic Movement.]
22. Ibid [Bye-Law to Rule 16–2.3.4 In evaluating candidatures linked to a function within an IF or NOC, the IOC Members Election Commission shall also take into consideration whether a candidate's respective IF or NOC has an athletes' commission which is compliant with the applicable regulations of the IOC, and that such IF or NOC is compliant with the Olympic Charter and the World Anti-Doping Code.]
23. Ibid [7. The IOC Medical and Scientific Commission: 7.1 The President establishes a Medical and Scientific Commission, the terms of reference of which shall include the following duties: 7.1.1 to implement the World Anti-Doping Code and all other IOC Anti-Doping Rules, in particular upon the occasion of the Olympic Games; 7.1.2 to elaborate guidelines relating to the medical care and health of the athletes; 7.2 Members of the Medical and Scientific Commission shall not act in any medical capacity whatsoever for the delegation of an NOC at the Olympic Games

nor participate in the discussions relating to non-compliance with the World Anti-Doping Code by members of their respective NOC's delegations.]

24. Ibid [27 Mission and role of the NOCs 2. The NOCs' role is: . . . 2.6 to adopt and implement the World Anti-Doping Code. . .]

25. Ibid [II. Participation in the Olympic Games 40 Participation in the Olympic Games* To participate in the Olympic Games, a competitor, team official or other team personnel must respect and comply with the Olympic Charter and World Anti-Doping Code, including the conditions of participation established by the IOC, as well as with the rules of the relevant IF as approved by the IOC, and the competitor, team official or other team personnel must be entered by his NOC.]

26. Ibid [Bye-Law to Rule 44–4. As a condition precedent to participation in the Olympic Games, every competitor shall comply with all the provisions of the Olympic Charter and the rules of the IF governing his sport. The NOC which enters the competitor is responsible for ensuring that such competitor is fully aware of and complies with the Olympic Charter and the World Anti-Doping Code . . . 6. All participants in the Olympic Games in whatever capacity must comply with the entry process as prescribed by the IOC Executive Board, including the signing of the entry form, which includes an obligation to (i) comply with the Olympic Charter and the World Anti-Doping Code and (ii) submit disputes to CAS jurisdiction. 45 Programme of the Olympic Games- . . . 3. The programme is established following a review by the IOC of the programme of the previous corresponding edition of the Olympic Games. Only sports which comply with the Olympic Charter and the World Anti-Doping Code are eligible to be in the programme . . . Bye-law to Rule 45–3.3. The Session is entitled to exclude from the programme any sport, at any time, if the relevant IF governing such sport does not comply with the Olympic Charter or the World Anti-Doping Code . . . 59 Measures and sanctions* In the case of any violation of the Olympic Charter, the World Anti-Doping Code, the Olympic Movement Code on the Prevention of Manipulation of Competitions or any other regulation, the measures or sanctions which may be taken by the Session, the IOC Executive Board or the disciplinary commission . . . 2. In the context of the Olympic Games, in the case of any violation of the Olympic Charter, of the World Anti-Doping Code, . . . 60 Challenging IOC decisions Notwithstanding the applicable rules and deadlines for all arbitration and appeal procedures, and subject to any other provision of the World Anti-Doping Code, no decision taken by the IOC concerning an edition of the Olympic Games, including but not limited to competitions and their consequences such as rankings or results, can be challenged by anyone after a period of three years from the day of the closing ceremony of such Games.]

27. World Anti-Doping Agency (n 1) [20.1.12 To cooperate with relevant national organizations and agencies and other Anti-Doping Organizations. 20.1.13 To respect the operational independence of laboratories as provided in the International Standard for Laboratories. 20.1.14 To adopt a policy or rule implementing Article 2.11.]

28. Ibid [20.7 Roles and Responsibilities of WADA]

29. Ibid [20.7.1 To accept the Code and commit to fulfill its roles and responsibilities under the Code through a declaration approved by WADA's Foundation Board.]

30. Ibid [20.7.2 To adopt and implement policies and procedures which conform with the Code and the International Standards.]

31. World Anti-Doping Agency (n 1) [20.7.3 To provide support and guidance to Signatories in their efforts to comply with the Code and the International Standards and monitor such compliance in accordance with Article 24.1 of the Code and the International Standard for Code Compliance by Signatories.]

32. Ibid [20.7.4 To approve International Standards applicable to the implementation of the Code.]

33. Ibid [20.7.5 To accredit and reaccredit laboratories to conduct Sample analysis or to approve others to conduct Sample analysis.]
34. Lovely Dasgupta, *The World Anti-Doping Code-Fit for Purpose?* (Routledge, 2019)
35. World Anti-Doping Agency (n 1) [20.7.6 To develop and publish guidelines and models of best practice.]
36. Ibid [20.7.7 To submit to the WADA Executive Committee for approval, upon the recommendation of the WADA Athletes Committee the Athletes' Anti-Doping Rights Act which compiles in one place those Athletes' rights which are specifically identified in the Code and International Standards, and other agreed upon principles of best practice with respect to the overall protection of Athletes' rights in the context of anti-doping.]
37. World Anti-Doping Agency, "Anti-Doping Rights Act Athletes' Play True [Approved by WADA's Executive Committee on 7 November 2019.] www.wada-ama.org/sites/default/files/resources/files/athlete_act_en.pdf (accessed 25th February 2021)
38. World Anti-Doping Agency (n 1) [20.7.8 To promote, conduct, commission, fund and coordinate anti-doping research and to promote anti-doping Education.]
39. Ibid [20.7.9 To design and conduct an effective Independent Observer Program and other types of Event advisory programs.]
40. Ibid [20.7.10 To conduct, in exceptional circumstances and at the direction of the WADA Director General, Testing on its own initiative or as requested by other Anti-Doping Organizations, and to cooperate with relevant national and international organizations and agencies, including but not limited to, facilitating inquiries and investigations.]
41. Ibid [To approve, in consultation with International Federations, National Anti-Doping Organizations, and Major Event Organizations, defined Testing and Sample analysis programs.]
42. Ibid [20.7.12 Subject to applicable law, as a condition of such position or involvement, to require all of its board members, directors, officers, and those employees (and those of appointed Delegated Third Parties), who are involved in any aspect of Doping Control, to agree to be bound by antidoping rules as Persons in conformity with the Code for direct and intentional misconduct, or to be bound by comparable rules and regulations put in place by the Signatory.]
43. Ibid [0.7.13 Subject to applicable law, to not knowingly employ a Person in any position involving Doping Control (other than authorized anti-doping Education or rehabilitation programs) who is Provisionally Suspended or is serving a period of Ineligibility under the Code or, if a Person was not subject to the Code, who has directly and intentionally engaged in conduct within the previous six (6) years which would have constituted a violation of anti-doping rules if Code-compliant rules had been applicable to such Person.]
44. World Anti-Doping Agency, "Intelligence and Investigations" www.wada-ama.org/en/what-we-do/intelligence-and-investigations (accessed 25th February 2021)
45. World Anti-Doping Agency (n 1) [20.7.14 To initiate its own investigations of anti-doping rule violations, non-compliance of Signatories and WADA-accredited laboratories, and other activities that may facilitate doping.]
46. Henning Eichberg, "Pyramid or Democracy in Sports? Alternative Ways in European Sports Policies" www.idrottsforum.org/articles/eichberg/eichberg080206.pdf (accessed 25th February 2021)
47. Tien-Chin Tan, Alan Bairner and Yu-Wen Chen, "Managing Compliance with the World Anti-Doping Code: China's Strategies and Their Implications" https://journals.sagepub.com/doi/abs/10.1177/1012690218805402 (accessed 25th February 2021)

48. World Anti-Doping Agency (n 1) [24.1 Monitoring and Enforcing Compliance with the Code- 24.1.1 Compliance by Signatories with the Code and the International Standards shall be monitored by WADA in accordance with the International Standard for Code Compliance by Signatories.]
49. Ibid [24.1.2: To facilitate such monitoring, each Signatory shall report to WADA on its compliance with the Code and the International Standards as and when required by WADA. As part of that reporting, the Signatory shall accurately provide all of the information requested by WADA and shall explain the actions it is taking to correct any Non-Conformities.]
50. Ibid [24.1.3 Failure by a Signatory to provide accurate information in accordance with Article 24.1.2 itself constitutes an instance of Non-Conformity with the Code, as does failure by a Signatory to submit accurate information to WADA where required by other Articles of the Code or by the International Standard for Code Compliance by Signatories or other International Standard.]
51. World Anti-Doping Agency (n 1) [24.1.4 In cases of Non-Conformity (whether with reporting obligations or otherwise), WADA shall follow the corrective procedures set out in the International Standard for Code Compliance by Signatories. If the Signatory or its delegate fails to correct the Non-Conformities within the specified timeframe, then (following approval of such course by WADA's Executive Committee) WADA shall send a formal notice to the Signatory, alleging that the Signatory is non-compliant, specifying the consequences that WADA proposes should apply for such non-compliance from the list of potential consequences set forth in Article 24.1.12, and specifying the conditions that WADA proposes the Signatory should have to satisfy in order to be Reinstated to the list of Code compliant Signatories. That notice will be publicly reported in accordance with the International Standard for Code Compliance by Signatories.]
52. Ibid [24.1.5 If the Signatory does not dispute WADA's allegation of non-compliance or the consequences or Reinstatement conditions proposed by WADA within twenty-one (21) days of receipt of the formal notice, the non-compliance alleged will be deemed admitted and the consequences and Reinstatement conditions proposed will be deemed accepted, the notice will automatically become and will be issued by WADA as a final decision, and (without prejudice to any appeal filed in accordance with Article 13.6) it will be enforceable with immediate effect in accordance with Article 24.1.9. The decision will be publicly reported as provided in the International Standard for Code Compliance by Signatories or other International Standards.]
53. Ibid [24.1.6 If the Signatory wishes to dispute WADA's allegation of non-compliance, and/or the consequences and/or the Reinstatement conditions proposed by WADA, it must notify WADA in writing within twenty-one (21) days of its receipt of the notice from WADA. In that event, WADA shall file a formal notice of dispute with CAS, and that dispute will be resolved by the CAS Ordinary Arbitration Division in accordance with the International Standard for Code Compliance by Signatories. WADA shall have the burden of proving to the CAS Panel, on the balance of probabilities, that the Signatory is non-compliant (if that is disputed). If the CAS Panel decides that WADA has met that burden, and if the Signatory has also disputed the consequences and/or the Reinstatement conditions proposed by WADA, the CAS Panel will also decide, by reference to the relevant provisions of the International Standard for Code Compliance by Signatories: (a) what consequences should be imposed from the list of potential consequences set out in Article 24.1.12 of the Code; and (b) what conditions the Signatory should be required to satisfy in order to be Reinstated.]
54. Ibid [24.1.7 WADA will publicly report the fact that the case has been referred to CAS for determination. Each of the following Persons shall have the right to

intervene and participate as a party in the case, provided it gives notice of its intervention within ten (10) days of such publication by WADA: 24.1.7.1 the International Olympic Committee and/or the International Paralympic Committee (as applicable), and the National Olympic Committee and/or the National Paralympic Committee (as applicable), where the decision may have an effect in relation to the Olympic Games or Paralympic Games (including decisions affecting eligibility to attend/ participate in the Olympic Games or Paralympic Games); and 24.1.7.2 an International Federation, where the decision may have an effect on participation in the International Federation's World Championships and/or other International Events and/ or on a bid that has been submitted for a country to host the International Federation's World Championships and/ or other International Events. Any other Person wishing to participate as a party in the case must apply to CAS within ten (10) days of publication by WADA of the fact that the case has been referred to CAS for determination. CAS shall permit such intervention (i) if all other parties in the case agree; or (ii) if the applicant demonstrates a sufficient legal interest in the outcome of the case to justify its participation as a party.]

55. World Anti-Doping Agency (n 1) [24.1.8 CAS's decision resolving the dispute will be publicly reported by CAS and by WADA. Subject to the right under Swiss law to challenge that decision before the Swiss Federal Tribunal, the decision shall be final and enforceable with immediate effect in accordance with Article 24.1.9.]

56. Ibid [24.1.9 Final decisions issued in accordance with Article 24.1.5 or Article 24.1.8, determining that a Signatory is non-compliant, imposing consequences for such non-compliance, and/ or setting conditions that the Signatory has to satisfy in order to be Reinstated to the list of Code-compliant Signatories, and decisions by CAS further to Article 24.1.10, are applicable worldwide, and shall be recognized, respected and given full effect by all other Signatories in accordance with their authority and within their respective spheres of responsibility.]

57. Ibid [24.1.10 If a Signatory wishes to dispute WADA's allegation that the Signatory has not yet met all of the Reinstatement conditions imposed on it and therefore is not yet entitled to be Reinstated to the list of Code-compliant Signatories, the Signatory must advise WADA in writing within twenty-one (21) days of its receipt of the allegation from WADA. In that event, WADA shall file a formal notice of dispute with CAS, and the dispute will be resolved by the CAS Ordinary Arbitration Division in accordance with Articles 24.1.6 to 24.1.8. WADA shall have the burden to prove to the CAS ARTICLE 24 Monitoring and Enforcing Compliance with the Code and UNESCO Convention World Anti-Doping Code 2021 151 ARTICLE 24 Monitoring and Enforcing Compliance with the Code and UNESCO Convention Panel, on the balance of probabilities, that the Signatory has not yet met all of the Reinstatement conditions imposed on it and therefore is not yet entitled to be Reinstated. Subject to the right under Swiss law to challenge CAS's decision before the Swiss Federal Tribunal, CAS's decision shall be final and enforceable with immediate effect in accordance with Article 24.1.9.]

58. Ibid [24.1.11 The various requirements imposed on Signatories by the Code and the International Standards shall be classified either as Critical, or as High Priority, or as General, in accordance with the International Standard for Code Compliance by Signatories, depending on their relative importance to the fight against doping in sport. That classification shall be a key factor in determining what consequences should be imposed in the event of non-compliance with such requirement(s), in accordance with Article 10 of the International Standard for Code Compliance by Signatories. The Signatory has the right to dispute the classification of the requirement, in which case CAS will decide on the appropriate classification.]

59. Ibid [24.1.12 The following consequences may be imposed, individually or cumulatively, on a Signatory that has failed to comply with the Code and/or the

International Standards, based on the particular facts and circumstances of the case at hand, and the provisions of Article 10 of the International Standard for Code Compliance by Signatories: 24.1.12.1 Ineligibility or withdrawal of WADA privileges: (a) in accordance with the relevant provisions of WADA's Statutes, the Signatory's Representatives being ruled ineligible for a specified period to hold any WADA office or any position as a member of any WADA board or committee or other body (including but not limited to WADA's Foundation Board, the Executive Committee, and any Standing Committee) (although WADA may exceptionally permit Representatives of the Signatory to remain as members of WADA expert groups where there is no effective substitute available).]

60. Ibid [(b) the Signatory being ruled ineligible to host any event organized or co-hosted or co-organized by WADA.]

61. World Anti-Doping Agency (n 1) [(c) the Signatory's Representatives being ruled ineligible to participate in any WADA Independent Observer Program or WADA Outreach program or other WADA activities.]

62. Ibid [(d) withdrawal of WADA funding to the Signatory (whether direct or indirect) relating to the development of specific activities or participation in specific programs.]

63. Ibid [24.1.12.2 the Signatory's Representatives being ruled ineligible for a specified period to hold any office of or position as a member of the board or committees or other bodies of any other Signatory (or its members) or association of Signatories.]

64. Ibid [24.1.12.3 Special Monitoring of some or all of the Signatory's Anti-Doping Activities, until WADA considers that the Signatory is in a position to implement such Anti-Doping Activities in a compliant manner without such monitoring.]

65. Ibid [24.1.12.4 Supervision and/or Takeover of some or all of the Signatory's Anti-Doping Activities by an Approved Third Party, until WADA considers that the Signatory is in a position to implement such Anti-Doping Activities itself in a compliant manner without such measures: (a) If the non-compliance involves non-compliant rules, regulations and/or legislation, then the Anti-Doping Activities in issue shall be conducted under other applicable rules (of one or more other Anti-Doping Organizations, e.g., International Federations or National Anti-Doping Organizations or Regional Anti-Doping Organizations) that are compliant, as directed by WADA. In that case, while the Anti-Doping Activities (including any Testing and Results Management) will be administered by the Approved Third Party under and in accordance with those other applicable rules at the cost of the non-compliant Signatory, any costs incurred by the Anti-Doping Organizations as a result of the use of their rules in this manner shall be reimbursed by the noncompliant Signatory. (b) If it is not possible to fill the gap in the Signatory's Anti-Doping Activities in this way (for example, because national legislation prohibits it, and the National Anti-Doping Organization has not secured an amendment to that legislation or other solution), then it may be necessary as an alternative measure to exclude Athletes who would have been covered by the Signatory's Anti-Doping Activities from participating in the Olympic Games/Paralympic Games/other Events, in order to protect the rights of clean Athletes and to preserve public confidence in the integrity of competition at those events.]

66. Ibid [24.1.12.5 A Fine.]

67. Ibid [24.1.12.6 Suspension or loss of eligibility to receive some or all funding and/or other benefits from the International Olympic Committee or the International Paralympic Committee or any other Signatory for a specified period (with or without the right to receive such funding and/or other benefits for that period retrospectively following Reinstatement).]

68. Ibid [Recommendation to the relevant public authorities to withhold some or all public and/or other funding and/or other benefits from the Signatory for a specified

period (with or without the right to receive such funding and/or other benefits for that period retrospectively following Reinstatement).]

69. Ibid [24.1.12.8 Where the Signatory is a National Anti-Doping Organization or a National Olympic Committee acting as a National Anti-Doping Organization, the Signatory's country being ruled ineligible to host or co-host and/or to be awarded the right to host or co-host an International Event (e.g., Olympic Games, Paralympic Games, any other Major Event Organization's Event, World Championships, regional or continental championships, and/or any other International Event): (a) If the right to host or co-host a World Championship and/or other International Event(s) has already been awarded to the country in question, the Signatory that awarded that right must assess whether it is legally and practically possible to withdraw that right and re-assign the Event to another country. If it is legally and practically possible to do so, then the Signatory shall do so. (b) Signatories shall ensure that they have due authority under their statutes, rules and regulations, and/ or hosting agreements, to comply with this requirement (including a right in any hosting agreement to cancel the agreement without penalty where the relevant country has been ruled ineligible to host the Event).]

70. Ibid [24.1.12.9 Where the Signatory is a National Anti-Doping Organization or a National Olympic Committee or a National Paralympic Committee, exclusion of the following Persons from participation in or attendance at the Olympic Games and the Paralympic Games and/or other specified Events, World Championships, regional or continental championships and/or any other International Events for a specified period: (a) the National Olympic Committee and/ or the National Paralympic Committee of the Signatory's country; (b) the Representatives of that country and/or of the National Olympic Committee and/or the National Paralympic Committee of that country; and/or (c) the Athletes and Athlete Support Personnel affiliated to that country and/ or to the National Olympic Committee and/ or to the National Paralympic Committee and/or to the National Federation of that country.]

71. Ibid [24.1.12.10 Where the Signatory is an International Federation, exclusion of the following Persons from participation in or attendance at the Olympic Games and the Paralympic Games and/or other Events for a specified period: The Representatives of that International Federation and/or the Athletes and Athlete Support Personnel participating in the International Federation's sport (or in one or more disciplines of that sport).]

72. Ibid [24.1.12.11 Where the Signatory is a Major Event Organization: (a) Special Monitoring or Supervision or Takeover of the Major Event Organization's Anti-Doping Activities at the next edition(s) of its Event; and/or (b) Suspension or loss of eligibility to receive funding and other benefits from and/or the recognition/ membership/ patronage (as applicable) of the International Olympic Committee, the International Paralympic Committee, the Association of National Olympic Committees, or other patron body; and/or (c) loss of recognition of its Event as a qualifying event for the Olympic Games or the Paralympic Games.]

73. Ibid [24.1.12.12 Suspension of recognition by the Olympic Movement and/or of membership of the Paralympic Movement.]

74. Ibid [24.1.13 Other Consequences Governments and Signatories and associations of Signatories may impose additional consequences within their respective spheres of authority for non-compliance by Signatories, provided that this does not compromise or restrict in any way the ability to apply consequences in accordance with this Article 24.1.]

75. Ibid [13.6 Appeals from Decisions under Article 24.1 A notice that is not disputed and so becomes a final decision under Article 24.1, finding a Signatory noncompliant with the Code and imposing consequences for such non-compliance, as well as

conditions for Reinstatement of the Signatory, may be appealed to CAS as provided in the International Standard for Code Compliance by Signatories.]

76. World Anti-Doping Agency, "International Standard Code Compliance by Signatories" www.wada-ama.org/sites/default/files/resources/files/international_standard_isccs_2020.pdf (accessed 25th February 2021)

77. Ibid [The International Standard for Code Compliance by Signatories sets out: • the roles, responsibilities, and procedures of the different bodies involved in WADA's compliance monitoring function (Part Two, Article 5); • the support and assistance that WADA will offer to Signatories in their efforts to comply with the Code and the International Standards (Part Two, Article 6); • the means by which WADA will monitor compliance by Signatories with their obligations under the Code and the International Standards (Part Two, Article 7); • the opportunities and support that WADA will offer to Signatories to correct Non-Conformities before any formal action is taken (Part Two, Article 8); • if a Signatory fails to correct the Non-Conformities, the process to be followed to get CAS to hear and determine an allegation of non-compliance and to determine the Signatory Consequences of such non-compliance. This process mirrors, insofar as is appropriate and practicable, the process followed in determining Code non-compliance and the Consequences of such non-compliance for Athletes and other Persons (Part Two, Articles 9 and 10; Annexes A and B); • the principles to be applied by CAS to determine the Signatory Consequences to be imposed in a particular case, depending on the facts and circumstances of that case (Part Two, Article 10; Annexes A and B); the procedures that WADA will follow to ensure that a Signatory that has been determined to be non-compliant, is Reinstated as quickly as possible once it has corrected that non-compliance (Part Two, Article 11); and • the transitional provisions applicable to proceedings pending as of 1 January 2021 (Part Two, Article 12).]

78. Ibid [5.0 Roles, Responsibilities and Procedures of the Different Bodies Involved in WADA's Compliance Monitoring Function.]

79. Ibid [5.2 Independent Review and Recommendations 5.2.1 The Compliance Review Committee is an independent, non-political WADA Standing Committee that oversees WADA's Code Compliance monitoring efforts and enforcement activities, and provides advice and recommendations on such matters to WADA's Executive Committee. 5.2.1.1 The CRC is governed by Terms of Reference designed to ensure the independence, political neutrality and specialization of its members that underpin the credibility of its work. The Terms of Reference include strict conflict of interest provisions that require CRC members to declare any potential conflicts of interest and to exclude themselves from all CRC deliberations in any matter in which they may have a conflict of interest. 5.2.2 The CRC follows standardized procedures encompassing review, assessment, communication, and the making of recommendations to WADA's Executive Committee on matters relating to Code Compliance, correction of Non-Conformities, and Reinstatement. These procedures (see Articles 8, 9 and 11) are designed to support a transparent, objective, and consistent approach to the assessment and enforcement of Code Compliance. 5.2.2.1 Where WADA Management reports apparent Non-Conformities to the CRC, a procedure is followed that gives the Signatory in question the time and opportunity to explain and correct the Non-Conformities within a specified timeframe as to achieve full Code Compliance (see Article 8). 5.2.2.2 If the Signatory does not correct the Non-Conformities within the framework of that procedure, the CRC will review the case in detail and decide whether to recommend to WADA's Executive Committee that a formal notice be issued to the Signatory alleging non-compliance (see Article 5.3). 5.2.3 In addition to reviewing and assessing compliance-related issues raised by WADA Management, at any time the CRC may identify compliance-related issues of its own accord to be addressed by WADA Management.]

80. Ibid [5.4 The Principle of Last Resort 5.4.1 Consistent with the principle of 'last resort', in any case (including not only ordinary but also fast track cases), if a Signatory does not meet the required timeframes for correcting Non-Conformities and so the case is referred to the CRC and beyond, provided that the Signatory corrects the Non-Conformities at any time before Signatory Consequences are imposed by CAS, then no Signatory Consequences shall be imposed, save to the extent that (a) costs have been incurred in pursuing the case before CAS (in which case the Signatory must cover those costs); and/or (b) the failure to correct a Non-Conformity within the required timeframe has resulted in irreparable prejudice to the fight against doping in sport (in which case Signatory Consequences may be imposed to reflect that prejudice).]
81. Ibid [5.5 Reinstatement Procedures.]
82. Ibid [6.0 WADA's Support for Signatories' Efforts to Achieve/Maintain Code Compliance.]
83. Ibid [7.0 Monitoring Signatories' Code Compliance Efforts 7.1 Objective 7.1.1 In accordance with its obligation under Code Articles 20.7.3 and 24.1.1 to monitor Code Compliance by Signatories, WADA reviews Signatories' rules and regulations (and/or legislation, if that is how the Code has been implemented in a particular country) to ensure that they are compliant with the Code and the International Standards. It also assesses whether Signatories are implementing their rules, regulations and legislation through Anti-Doping Programs that meet all of the requirements of the Code and the International Standards. The purpose of Article 7 is to set out the standards that will govern these monitoring activities. The objective will always be to make the monitoring process as efficient and cost-effective as possible.]
84. Ibid [7.2 Prioritization Between Different Signatories . . . 7.2.2 Given the large number of Signatories and WADA's limited resources, the CRC may approve proposals by WADA Management to prioritize the monitoring for Code Compliance (a) of certain categories of Signatories, based on the scope of the AntiDoping Activities required of such categories of Signatories under the Code; and/ or (b) of certain specific Signatories, based on an objective Risk Assessment. The following is a non-exhaustive list of factors that may be considered in such an assessment: 7.2.2.1 (where the Signatory is an International Federation) the physiological risk of doping in a particular sport/discipline; 7.2.2.2 (where the Signatory is an International Federation) participation of the Signatory in the Olympic and/or Paralympic Games; 7.2.2.3 (where the Signatory is a Major Event Organization) the level of Athletes participating in the Event; 7.2.2.4 performances by Athletes from a particular country in International Events; 7.2.2.5 a history of doping in a particular country or a particular sport/discipline; 7.2.2.6 a Signatory's response to a Mandatory Information Request or a Code Compliance Questionnaire; 7.2.2.7 receipt of credible intelligence or the results of an investigation suggesting there may be significant Non-Conformities in the Signatory's Anti-Doping Program; 7.2.2.8 a Signatory's breach of Critical or High Priority requirements under the Code or an International Standard; 7.2.2.9 a Signatory's failure to implement recommendations following collaboration programs in which WADA acted as a facilitator or a party; 7.2.2.10 a Signatory's failure to implement measures (e.g., Target Testing) following a recommendation made or endorsed by WADA (e.g., in relation to Testing in the lead-up to the Olympic Games or Paralympic Games or other Event); 7.2.2.11 (where the Signatory is a NADO or a National Olympic Committee acting as a NADO) the fact that the Signatory's country hosts a WADA-accredited laboratory and/or is bidding to host or has won the right to host a major sporting event; 7.2.2.12 where a Signatory that has been found to be non-compliant is seeking to be Reinstated; and/or

7.2.2.13 a request by WADA's Executive Committee and/or WADA's Foundation Board.]

85. Ibid [7.2.4 In addition, again given the large number of Signatories and WADA's limited resources, the CRC may approve proposals by WADA Management to prioritize enforcement of Critical and (in certain circumstances) High Priority requirements of the Code and/or the International Standards (including, where necessary, by alleging non-compliance and proposing imposition of Signatory Consequences), while giving Signatories additional opportunity to take any corrective action(s) necessary to ensure compliance with other requirements of the Code and/or the International Standards. The greatest priority will be given to pursuing the imposition of appropriate Signatory Consequences in cases involving non-compliance with Critical requirements and Aggravating Factors.]

86. Ibid [7.4 WADA's Monitoring Tools]

87. Ibid [7.6 Mandatory Information Requests 7.6.1 Independent of any other monitoring activity, where WADA receives or collects information indicating that a Signatory may not be complying with Critical or High Priority requirements, WADA Management may send the Signatory a Mandatory Information Request requiring it to provide information that enables WADA to confirm the actual position. WADA shall only request information that is necessary for WADA to assess the Signatory's Code Compliance effectively, and that is not already available to WADA through other sources (such as ADAMS). The request will explain why WADA Management is asking for the information and will specify the date for the Signatory to provide it (which date shall be no less than twenty-one (21) days later). 7.6.2 WADA Management will assign a WADA Auditor to review the response received from the Signatory and to provide an assessment and recommendation, including (where appropriate) a recommendation to issue a Corrective Action Report in accordance with Article 8.2.2.7.6.3. If the Signatory fails to provide the required response to a Mandatory Information Request by the date that WADA has specified for receipt of such response, that will trigger the process outlined in Article 8.3.1.]

88. Ibid [7.7 The Compliance Audit Program]

89. World Anti-Doping Agency (n 76) [7.8 Continuous Compliance Monitoring 7.8.1 WADA Management will identify a number of requirements (in consultation with the CRC) for which Signatories will be subject to continuous compliance monitoring, using means that are complementary to the Code Compliance Questionnaire and Compliance Audits.]

90. Ibid [7.9 Special Provisions Applicable to Major Event Organizations 7.9.1 Major Event Organizations are subject to the same Code Compliance monitoring and enforcement rules and procedures set out in this International Standard for Code Compliance by Signatories as all other Signatories. However, Major Event Organizations may also be made the subject of an Independent Observer Program; and the normal procedures for identification and correction of Non-Conformities may have to be fast-tracked for them, in the manner set out in this Article 7.9, due to the timing of their Events. For the avoidance of doubt, unless otherwise stated in this Article 7.9, the normal rules, procedures and timeframes set out in this International Standard for Code Compliance by Signatories shall apply to Major Event Organizations. . .]

91. Ibid [8.0 Giving Signatories the Opportunity to Correct Non-Conformities 8.1 Objective 8.1.1 When Non-Conformities are identified, the objective will be to assist the Signatory through dialogue and support to correct the Non-Conformities and so achieve and maintain full Code Compliance. 8.1.2 Article 8 sets out the procedures that WADA will follow in giving the Signatory adequate opportunity to correct the Non-Conformities identified.]

92. Ibid [8.4 Referral to the CRC]

93. Ibid [9.0 Confirming Non-Compliance and Imposing Signatory Consequences 9.1 CRC Recommendation 9.1.1 Articles 8.4 and 8.5 identify the circumstances in which the CRC may recommend that the Signatory be sent a formal notice alleging non-compliance with the requirements of the Code and/or the International Standards, categorizing the requirements in question as Critical, High Priority, or General, identifying any Aggravating Factors alleged by WADA (in cases involving non-compliance with Critical requirements), specifying the Signatory Consequences that it is contended should apply for such noncompliance (in accordance with Article 10), and specifying the conditions that it is proposed the Signatory should have to satisfy in order to be Reinstated (in accordance with Article 11).]
94. Ibid [9.2 Consideration by WADA's Executive Committee]
95. Ibid [9.3 Acceptance by the Signatory; 9.4 Determination by CAS]
96. Ibid [9.4.3 Consistent with the principle of 'last resort', in any case (including not only ordinary but also fast track cases), if a Signatory does not meet the required timeframes for correcting Non-Conformities, and therefore the case is referred to the CRC, if the Signatory corrects the Non-Conformities to the satisfaction of the CRC at any time before Signatory Consequences are imposed by CAS, then it will avoid any such Signatory Consequences, save to the extent that costs have been incurred in pursuing the case before CAS (in which case the Signatory must cover those costs) and/or the failure to correct a Non-Conformity within the required timeframe has resulted in irreparable prejudice (in which case Signatory Consequences may be imposed to reflect that prejudice).]
97. Ibid [10.2 Principles Relevant to the Determination of the Signatory Consequences to be Applied in a Particular Case.]
98. Ibid [11.0 Reinstatement]
99. World Anti-Doping Agency (n 1)
100. World Anti-Doping Agency, "World Anti-Doping Program 2018 Anti-Doping Rule Violations (ADRVs) Report- {This Report Is Compiled Based on Decisions Received by WADA Before 2 March 2020}" www.wada-ama.org/sites/default/files/resources/files/2018_adrv_report.pdf (accessed 25th March 2021)
101. Ibid
102. World Anti-Doping Agency (n 1)
103. World Anti-Doping Agency (n 76)
104. CAS 2020/O/6689
105. Ibid
106. CAS 2020/O/6689 para 860
107. CAS 2020/A/6978 & CAS 2020/A/7068
108. Ibid para 12
109. World Anti-Doping Agency, "World Anti-Doping Code 2015 with 2019 Amendments" [10.5 Reduction of the Period of Ineligibility based on No Significant Fault or Negligence. 10.5.1.2 Contaminated Products In cases where the Athlete or other Person can establish No Significant Fault or Negligence and that the detected Prohibited Substance came from a Contaminated Product, then the period of Ineligibility shall be, at a minimum, a reprimand and no period of Ineligibility, and at a maximum, two years Ineligibility, depending on the Athlete's or other Person's degree of Fault. 10.5.2 Application of No Significant Fault or Negligence beyond the Application of Article 10.5.1. If an Athlete or other Person establishes in an individual case where Article 10.5.1 is not applicable, that he or she bears No Significant Fault or Negligence, then, subject to further reduction or elimination as provided in Article 10.6, the otherwise applicable period of Ineligibility may be reduced based on the Athlete or other Person's degree of Fault, but the reduced period of Ineligibility may not be less than one-half of the period of Ineligibility

otherwise applicable. If the otherwise applicable period of Ineligibility is a lifetime, the reduced period under this Article may be no less than eight years.]
110. CAS 2020/A/6978 & CAS 2020/A/7068 (n 107) para 138
111. Ibid para 139
112. CAS 2020/A/6978 & CAS 2020/A/7068 (n 107) 167
113. "Copenhagen Declaration on Anti-Doping in Sport of 3 March 2003" www. wada-ama.org/sites/default/files/resources/files/WADA_Copenhagen_Declaration_EN.pdf (accessed 25th February 2021)
114. "International Convention against Doping in Sport" https://en.unesco.org/themes/sport-and-anti-doping/convention (accessed 25th February 2021)
115. World Anti-Doping Agency (n 1) [Article 22 Involvement of Governments- . . . 22.9 Each government should not limit or restrict WADA's access to any doping Samples or anti-doping records or information held or controlled by any Signatory, member of a Signatory or WADA-accredited or approved laboratory. 22.10 Failure by a government to ratify, accept, approve, or accede to the UNESCO Convention may result in ineligibility to bid for and/or host Events as provided in Articles 20.1.11, 20.3.14, and 20.6.9, and the failure by a government to comply with the UNESCO Convention thereafter, as determined by UNESCO, may result in meaningful consequences by UNESCO and WADA as determined by each organization.]
116. Ibid [24.2 Monitoring Compliance with the UNESCO Convention Compliance with the commitments reflected in the UNESCO Convention will be monitored as determined by the Conference of Parties to the UNESCO Convention, following consultation with the State Parties and WADA. WADA shall advise governments on the implementation of the Code by the Signatories and shall advise Signatories on the ratification, acceptance, approval or accession to the UNESCO Convention by governments.]

References

- World Anti-Doping Agency, "World Anti-Doping Code 2021" www.wada-ama.org/sites/default/files/resources/files/2021_wada_code.pdf (accessed 21 February 2021)
- Richard Pound, "The Olympics and the Paradox of Commercialization" https://hbr.org/2012/08/the-olympics-and-the-paradox-o (accessed 25th February 2021)
- Travis Nelson, "Sport Without Referees? The Power of the International Olympic Committee and the Social Politics of Accountability" www.icsspe.org/system/files/Nelson%20%26%20Cottrell%20-%20Sport%20without%20referees%20-%20The%20power%20of%20the%20IOC%20and%20the%20social%20politiscs%20of%20accountability.pdf (accessed 25th February 2021)
- Jonathan Grix and Donna Lee, "Soft Power, Sports Mega-Events and Emerging States: The Lure of the Politics of Attraction" www.tandfonline.com/doi/pdf/10.1080/13600826.2013.827632 (accessed 25th February 2021)
- World Anti-Doping Agency, "Independent Observer Program" www.wada-ama.org/en/what-we-do/independent-observer-program (accessed 25th February 2021)
- IOC—Greg Martin, "Pre-Games Anti-Doping Programme for Tokyo 2020 to Be the Most Extensive Ever" www.olympic.org/news/pre-games-anti-doping-programme-for-tokyo-2020-to-be-the-most-extensive-ever (accessed 25th February 2021)
- Lovely Dasgupta, *The World Anti-Doping Code-Fit for Purpose?* (Routledge, 2019)
- World Anti-Doping Agency, "Anti-Doping Rights Act Athletes' Play True [Approved by WADA's Executive Committee on 7 November 2019]" www.wada-ama.org/sites/default/files/resources/files/athlete_act_en.pdf (accessed 25th February 2021)

- World Anti-Doping Agency, "Intelligence and Investigations" www.wada-ama.org/en/what-we-do/intelligence-and-investigations (accessed 25th February 2021)
- Henning Eichberg, "Pyramid or Democracy in Sports? Alternative Ways in European Sports Policies" www.idrottsforum.org/articles/eichberg/eichberg080206.pdf (accessed 25th February 2021)
- Tien-Chin Tan, Alan Bairner and Yu-Wen Chen, "Managing Compliance with the World Anti-Doping Code: China's Strategies and Their Implications" https://journals.sagepub.com/doi/abs/10.1177/1012690218805402 (accessed 25th February 2021)
- World Anti-Doping Agency, "International Standard Code Compliance by Signatories" www.wada-ama.org/sites/default/files/resources/files/international_standard_isccs_2020.pdf (accessed 25th February 2021)
- World Anti-Doping Agency, "World Anti-Doping Program 2018 Anti-Doping Rule Violations (ADRVs) Report- {This Report Is Compiled Based on Decisions Received by WADA Before 2 March 2020}" www.wada-ama.org/sites/default/files/resources/files/2018_adrv_report.pdf (accessed 25th March 2021)
- CAS 2020/O/6689
- "Copenhagen Declaration on Anti-Doping in Sport of 3 March 2003" www.wada-ama.org/sites/default/files/resources/files/WADA_Copenhagen_Declaration_EN.pdf (accessed 25th February 2021)
- "International Convention Against Doping in Sport" https://en.unesco.org/themes/sport-and-anti-doping/convention (accessed 25th February 2021)

7 Epilogue

The Non-Olympic sport, with the doping cases score in single digit, needs to catch up with the Olympic sport in terms of compliance. And that can only be achieved if they seamlessly integrate within the compliance system of the WADA Code. However, the WADA Code has not incorporated any provision to ensure this integration. The role of ARISF is important in insisting on more rigorous monitoring of the compliance by the Non-Olympic sport. The ARISF needs to take a leaf out of the book of the Olympic sport. There has to be proper scrutiny before a sport is admitted as a member of the ARISF. Further, the ARISF should coordinate with the IOC to have proper screening before a sport is recognized. To insist on WADA Code compliance as a condition precedent to recognition of a sport by the IOC is problematic. This is so because such an insistence does not take into account the lack of monitoring to ensure actual compliance. In the absence of such monitoring, a sport just has to put in place formal compliance measures. IOC, without having any clear guidelines as to such monitoring, grants recognition based on the proof of formal compliance. Hence, there is a failure of monitoring at the pre-recognition stage. As the case load reveals even at the postrecognition stage, there are no strict compliances on the part of the Non-Olympic sport. Consequently, the insistence on WADA Code compliance by the IOC remains in letter but not in spirit. It becomes mere paperwork without having any real-time impact on the Non-Olympic sport. Further, such an insistence also has the potential of weakening the WADA Code and the entire anti-doping system. It also has the potential of increasing the burden on WADA to monitor sports at pre-recognition stage. And a failure to do the same will undermine the legitimacy of WADA. Hence, it is advisable to do away with the requirement of WAD Code compliance. As the review in the next few chapters will reveal, the Non-Olympic sport might not be amenable to strict WADA Code compliance. Hence in the interest of all the stakeholders, it is important that the requirement of the WADA Code compliance be revisited. IOC needs to do the same to strengthen WADA as well as the anti-doping movement.

One of the best examples which can be given to prove that the compliance laxity among the Non-Olympic sport undermines WADA is the American football. American football's evolution from an amateur activity to an excessively

DOI: 10.4324/9781003082309-7

commercialized entity is fascinating. The evolution, however, has not been smooth. At the same time, it has been a learning experience for the people in-charge of running the sport. The growth trajectory of the amateur and the professional version of the sport has had its effect on the response toward anti-doping measures. The amateur sports dreams of becoming an Olympic sport one day and thus they have promptly adopted the WADA Code. However, there is a symbiotic relationship that the amateur has with its professional counterpart. Hence, IFAF has naturally veered toward collaboration with NFL. The professional league, viz., NFL however has an anti-doping policy dictated by the CBG and it does not match the standards of the Code. Nonetheless, there continues to be a benign response from both the IOC and WADA toward this collaboration. And consequently, IFAF's collaboration with NFL grows from strength to strength. The non-acceptance of the Code by the NFL ought to have made IFAF terminate its association. However, IFAF is dictated by commercial incentives to support and promote NFL's games worldwide. Thus, the entire narrative of anti-doping regulation within the IFAF is dictated by the better bargaining power of NFL. And the benign response of IOC and WADA to IFAF's clear dereliction is governed by the greater bargaining power of the USA. Hence treatment of IFAF re-affirms the point that there is a clear disparity within the world of sports between Olympic and Non-Olympic sports. There is no parity or equality when it comes to applying and enforcing the anti-doping regulations among these two categories. The paragraphs hereunder establish this point.

WADA's legitimacy is also under attack in the game of cricket and it's just not cricket. The South Asian market of cricket is too big to be ignored and ICC realizes the same. Further, IPL has changed the narrative to an extent that it rivals all official matches in terms of popularity. Given this scenario, the acceptance of NADA by BCCI is indeed a great achievement for all concerned. However, one has to be skeptical about the fruitfulness of this development. A cursory look through BCCI's website does not reveal much. Importantly, the link to NADA has not yet been updated. It continues to take one to the 2015 WADA Code, as adopted by NADA. On the other hand, NADA has updated its Code version as well as the Prohibited list. The same is in compliance with the 2021 version. Further unlike the ICC website, BCCI does not have any information about the whereabouts filing or its procedure, as designed for the players. Importantly, there is no information that a person will get from the BCCI's webpage on Anti-Doping. It is as sparse as it can be and gives minimal information on the steps BCCI has taken or will take to ramp up the anti-doping measures. In so far as ICC is concerned its hand is clearly tied due to the financial incentive that BCCI provides. While on paper ICC appears to be taking steps for effective compliance, the same falls short of expected standards. And ICC's dilemma vis-à-vis BCCI is also reflective of the privilege that the Non-Olympic sport enjoys when it comes to WADA Code compliance. Hence, neither ICC nor BCCI is likely to face the heat from IOC or WADA for its poor record. And the fact that IOC continues to recognize ICC despite all the laxity on the part of its member NCF is revealing. The IOC too can wield the stick only if the sport is part of the Olympic program. And the ICC BCCI tussle exemplifies this as it has been seen in the case of IFAF and NFL. And this inherent dichotomy between Olympic and Non-Olympic sports vis-à-vis the anti-doping compliance continues to challenge the legitimacy of WADA Code.

A small IF of Dance sport, viz., WDSF too is lax in WADA Code compliance. The WDSF needs to take the matter of enforcement seriously for there are problems galore. Notwithstanding the fact that it has well-maintained website, the information on compliance is absolutely basic. Empirical studies done by researchers in the field of Dance sport and performance-enhancing drugs have found surprising information. It was found that substance abuse is most common among the athletes in Dance sports. The research found that the athletes rarely trust their coaches or physicians in the matter of doping. It was also found that female and young athletes are more prone to doping. It was also found that anti-doping education among the athletes involved in Dance sport is poor. These factors are some of many issues which WDSF needs to take note of before it aims to become an Olympic sport. Being one of the oldest Non-Olympic sport, it should have set its house in order. However, till date there are problems with respect to compliance with the WADA Code. Though the decisions delivered post 2015 appear to be better reasoned, it really does not help improve the argument of poor compliance. There is more than enough evidence that Dance sport like all others is prone to excessive doping. Dancers too need to boost stamina, heal injuries, and increase the level of Oxygen in their blood. They would need better genes to increase flexibility and agility in their body. They would need to improve their concentration. They would need to increase their power and boost their physique. In short, Dancers would need all that any other athlete would need. Hence, WDSF cannot push the issue of doping under the carpet. It needs to up the ante for its members and ensure that they enforce the WADA Code in the most stringent way. It needs to improve the anti-doping education and ensure that the elite-level player does not take medication without consulting qualified practitioners.

To treat Dance differently because it is an art as well as to create a false sense of confidence. Dance may be art as well but artists too can dope. Hence the fact that the art is also a sport and the WDSF is a signatory to WADA is a good enough reason to take doping seriously. The health reason of the athletes is a compelling issue as well for WDSF to take measures to check doping. Taking the athlete into confidence and constantly taking their feedback is needed to identify the loopholes in the compliance mechanism. Herein, WDSF needs to be pressurized by IOC and WADA. As stated again and again, the entire check and balance need to be done at the stage of granting recognition. Once the recognition is granted then the monitoring needs to be done diligently. Here, IOC needs to be proactive and seeks a report from the WDSF as to the measures taken to comply with the WADA Code. In addition, WADA too needs to play a proactive role in ensuring that the WDSF does not end up letting its athlete go scot-free. WDSF's website reveals tremendous growth and popularity of the sport. Hence, to argue that it is a small IF and hence has limited resources is not convincing. Importantly, WDSF can collaborate with WADA and IOC and discharge effectively its role as the enforcer of the WADA Code. Being a Non-Olympic sport and part of the Olympic system for long WDSF should understand the nuances of the anti-doping system. Being lax with the compliance, WDSF is also putting the players at risk of getting caught. It will also mean that the players are at the risk of losing their careers. Hence, as a Non-Olympic sport with the ambition of getting admitted to the Olympic Games, it needs to be serious about compliances with the WADA Code. However, the most important role needs to be played by IOC and WADA in ensuring compliances of the Non-Olympic sports.

Thus, one cannot but note that the Non-Olympic sports are a creation of the IOC. The recognition is granted by the IOC hence the liability to ensure Code compliance has to be on the IOC. Considering the excessive power that the Code has conferred on WADA, it too is equally responsible for the non-compliance of the Non-Olympic sports. In this set up, the State is just a bystander more so in a situation where the State has not contributed to the non-compliance. The Non-Olympic sports, not being part of the Olympic movement do not make the State realize their obligations under the WADA Code. Importantly, the State can only be made liable where it has aided or abetted a systemic doping. The State thus should be held liable when it has explicitly gone back in its commitment under the UNESCO Convention. And that should be limited to the Olympic sports for the State definitely has the duty to ensure that the IFs participating in Olympic program and IOC-recognized event are Code compliant. Importantly, since they are being sent on behalf of the National Olympic Committees which use the color and flag of the concerned State. In the case of Non-Olympic sports, such participation within the Olympic movement is missing. Non-Olympic sports are primarily confined to the competitions that their IFs organize. They may participate in multisport competitions where the Non-Olympic sports IF is a member. This clear demarcation between the status of Olympic sports as compared to the Non-Olympic sports is a ground that the States should be exempted. A Non-Olympic sports exemption ought to be created in favor of the State within the Code. As the State is not responsible if IOC and WADA, without applying any rigor, grant recognition to all and sundry. Any arm twisting in this regard of the State will be usurping their Sovereignty. The State should also not be liable in the case of those sports which do not depend on State funding for their existence. In such a case, even if the State allows its flag and logo to be used by such a sport it still does not bear responsibility. For the conduct is exclusive of the sport concerned and being a Code signatory they ought to on their own comply with WADA.

Index

For Product Safety Concerns and Information please contact our EU
representative GPSR@taylorandfrancis.com
Taylor & Francis Verlag GmbH, Kaufingerstraße 24, 80331 München, Germany

www.ingramcontent.com/pod-product-compliance
Lightning Source LLC
Chambersburg PA
CBHW060313220326
41598CB00027B/4314